Anatomy of Hearing and Speech

Anatomy of Hearing and Speech

Roderick P. Singh, Ph.D.
Health Sciences Centre
University of Western Ontario

New York Oxford
OXFORD UNIVERSITY PRESS
1980

Library of Congress Cataloging in Publication Data

Singh, Roderick P
Anatomy of hearing and speech.

Bibliography: p.
Includes index.
1. Larynx—Anatomy. 2. Ear—Anatomy.
3. Speech—Physiological aspects.
4. Hearing—Physiological aspects.
I. Title
QM255.S56 611'.9 79-19688
ISBN 0-19-502665-9 ISBN 0-19-502666-7 pbk.

Printed in the United States of America

Dedicated to my wife
Elizabeth,
to my children
Kristin, Kecia, and Kara,
and to the memory of
Uncle Joe

Preface

This volume contains basic information on the morphology of the anatomical structures associated with the organs of hearing and speech. It is primarily designed as a supplementary text for students enrolled in a communicative disorders program. However, it is also appropriate for students interested in vocal music, drama, or public speaking. Although a basic knowledge of anatomy is presupposed, a glossary of anatomical terms is included for the benefit of the student without a background in anatomy.

Anatomy is a visual subject, and numerous illustrations are included. These, however, should be supplemented by reference to the appropriate sections in comprehensive anatomy texts and atlases. If at all possible, the student should also examine museum specimens and models.

I am deeply indebted to many individuals who contributed to the completion of this work. Special appreciation is due Jane Vogan for her patience and skill in converting my amateurish sketches into accurate and professional illustrations and Callie Cesarini for her willing and efficient secretarial help. Finally, I would like to express my appreciation to the staff of Oxford University Press for their advice and assistance.

R. P. S.

Department of Anatomy
University of Western Ontario
London, Ontario
January, 1980

Contents

Illustrations

Figure

Tables

1
The Skeletal Framework

THE SKELETAL SYSTEM

The skeletal system may be described as a system of bones and related cartilage connected by articulations (joints). In human beings, the skeleton lies within the body, completely covered by soft tissue. Despite its appearance in museum specimens, bone is living, dynamic tissue and is capable of growth, adaptation, and regeneration. The chief functions of bones are:

1. *Support.* Bones serve as points of attachment for the soft tissues of the body.
2. *Protection.* The bones of the cranium protect the delicate brain tissue. The thoracic cage protects the heart and lungs.
3. *Hemopoiesis.* Red marrow, in which blood cell formation occurs, is found in the cavities of certain bones, for example, sternum, ribs, and proximal ends of the humerus and femur.

4. *Movement.* Bones serve as levers, and their articulations serve as fulcrums upon which muscles act.

There are approximately 215 bones in the human skeleton. Occasionally, this figure may vary as a result of the presence of extra sesamoid bones. The skeleton is usually divided into two parts: A. the axial skeleton, which comprises the bones of the head, neck, and trunk; and B. the appendicular skeleton, which comprises the bones of the limbs. The bones of the various parts of the body are summarized as follows:

A. **Axial skeleton**

1. Skull	22 bones
Cranium	8 bones
Facial skeleton and mandible	14 bones
2. Vertebral column	33 bones
Cervical vertebrae	7 bones
Thoracic vertebrae	12 bones
Lumbar vertebrae	5 bones
Sacral vertebrae	5 bones
Coccygeal vertebrae	4 bones

The sacral and coccygeal vertebrae are fused together to form the sacrum and coccyx, respectively.

3. Ribs (12 pairs)	24 bones
4. Sternum	1 bone

B. **Appendicular skeleton**

1. Upper limb	32 bones
Pectoral girdle—scapula and clavicle	2 bones
Humerus	1 bone
Radius and ulna	2 bones
Carpal bones (wrist)	8 bones
Metacarpal bones (hand)	5 bones
Phalangeal bones (hand)	14 bones

2. Lower limb	32 bones
Pelvic girdle Innominate or hip bones	2 bones
Femur	1 bone
Patella (knee cap)	1 bone
Tibia and fibula	2 bones
Tarsal bones (ankle)	7 bones
Metarsal bones (foot)	5 bones
Phalangeal bones (foot)	14 bones

There are seven other bones that are usually not regarded as part of the axial or appendicular skeleton. They are placed in a separate category—the visceral skeleton. These bones are the three ossicles of each ear and the hyoid bone.

For a detailed description of each bone of the skeleton, the student is referred to one of the many excellent texts available. As far as this text is concerned, the parts of the skeleton that are intimately related to the hearing and speech mechanism, such as the temporal bone and the thorax, will be described in detail in subsequent sections.

ARTICULATIONS

In order to enhance our understanding of the skeletal system, it is necessary to consider the ways in which bones are joined together or articulate with each other. Articulations may be classified either on the basis of degree of movement permitted, for example, immovable, slightly movable, or freely movable, or on a structural basis as fibrous, cartilaginous, or synovial. The following list combines both systems.

A. **Fibrous**—no joint cavity

1. Suture: synarthroses—minimal fibrous tissue present; immovable (e.g., joints between bones of vault of skull)
2. Syndesmosis: larger amount of fibrous tissue than above; slightly movable (e.g., radioulnar syndesmosis)

B. **Cartilaginous**—no joint cavity

1. Synchondrosis: slightly movable (e.g., ribs and costal cartilages)
2. Symphysis: slightly movable (e.g., joints between the bodies of the pubic bones)

C. **Synovial**—joint cavity present

All synovial joints are freely movable. A diagrammatic representation of a synovial joint is shown in Figure 1-1.

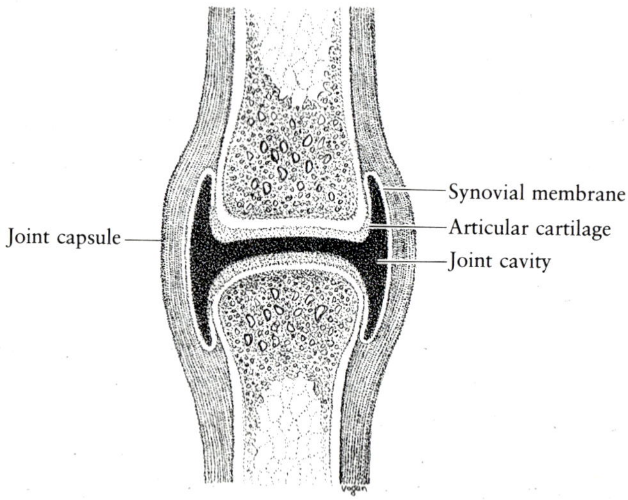

Figure 1-1. Synovial joint

1. Arthrodia (gliding)—articulating surfaces are small and flat or concave; one bone slides over the other (e.g., carpal bones)
2. Ginglymus (hinge)—movement in one plane at right angles to axis of bone (e.g., elbow, fingers)
3. Trochoid (pivot)—movement around one axis (e.g., radioulnar joint, atlas/axis joint)

4. Condyloid (ellipsoid)—biaxial—movement in two directions, (e.g., wrist)
5. Saddle—bones reciprocally concavoconvex, biaxial movement possible (e.g., carpometacarpal articulation of thumb)
6. Ball and socket—free movement in all planes (e.g., shoulder joint)

For the sake of completeness, the following structures, which are associated with joints, must be described.

1. *Bursa(e)* ("small purse"). This is a fibrous connective tissue sac filled with fluid similar to synovial fluid. It is usually found under muscles and tendons and serves as a protective device where these structures pass over bones. It permits easy movement of one part over another. Bursae may be in communication with the joint capsule, for example, suprapatellar bursa.
2. *Tendon sheaths.* These fibrous connective tissue sleeves containing a fluid similar to synovial fluid surround tendons as they pass over bones or run in bony canals. They reduce friction and protect the tendon, for example, the tendon of flexor muscles of fingers.

THE SKULL

In connection with the topics covered by this text, it is necessary to discuss the bones of the skull in some detail. The bones of the skull may be divided into two groups: A. the bones that enclose the brain and are referred to as the cranial bones, and B. the bones that make up the facial structures and are referred to as the facial bones. The mandible (lower jaw) will be included in this second group.

A. **Cranium**

The cranium is made up of eight bones as follows:

1. *Frontal bone.* This single bone makes up the anterosuperior part of the cranium (Figure 1-2). It articulates with the pari-

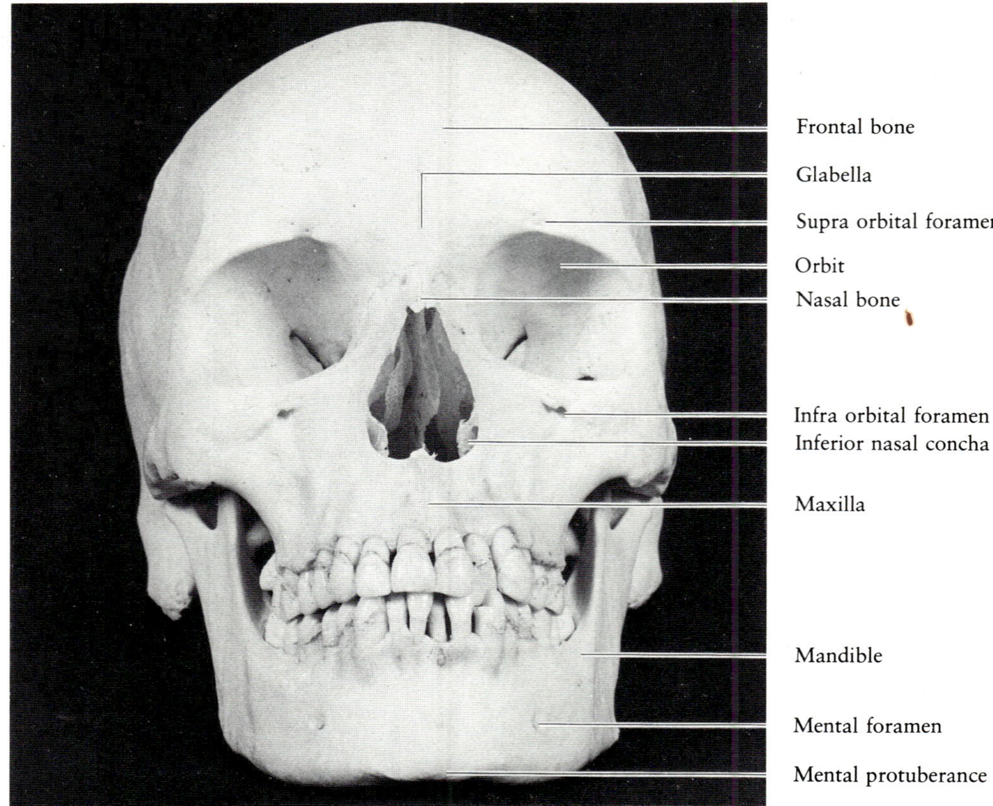

Figure 1-2. Skull—front view

etal bones at the coronal suture (Figure 1-3). Major landmarks on this bone are shown in Figure 1-2.

2. *Parietal bone* (paired). These bones make up the lateral and superior walls of the cranium. They articulate with the frontal, temporal, and occipital bones, as well as with each other at the sagittal suture (Figure 1-3).
3. Occipital bone. This single bone forms the posterobasal part of the cranium (Figure 1-4). It contains the foramen magnum.
4. Temporal bone (paired). These bones are located on the lateral side of the cranium (Figure 1-5). Embryologically, they arise from several separate primordia and, as a result, are usually described as consisting of four parts, namely squamous, tympanic, petromastoid, and styloid portions. It should be mentioned that the squamous and tympanic parts arise through membraneous ossification, whereas the petromastoid and styloid parts arise from cartilage precursors.
   a. *Squamous part.* The squamous portion is relatively thin and forms the anterior and upper part of the temporal bone. A slight depression seen on the lateral surface serves as the site of attachment of the temporalis muscle. Above the external auditory meatus is a small triangular depression called the suprameatal triangle. The mastoid anthrum lies medial to the suprameatal triangle. The suprameatal spine is a small projection below the suprameatal triangle. A major structure on the squamous part of the temporal bone is the zygomatic process.

      The zygomatic process has a somewhat triangular base just superior and anterior to the external auditory meatus. It extends forward to articulate with the temporal process of the zygomatic bone. The zygomatic process contributes, inferiorly, to the lateral part of the mandibular fossa. Anterior to the mandibular fossa is the articular tubercle, which is also involved in the temporomandibular joint. The remainder of the inferior surface provides attachment for the masseter muscle. The mandibular fossa has two parts: (i) an articular part that is a smooth and deeply concave depression on the inferior surface of the temporal bone, and (ii) a posterior, nonarticular surface formed

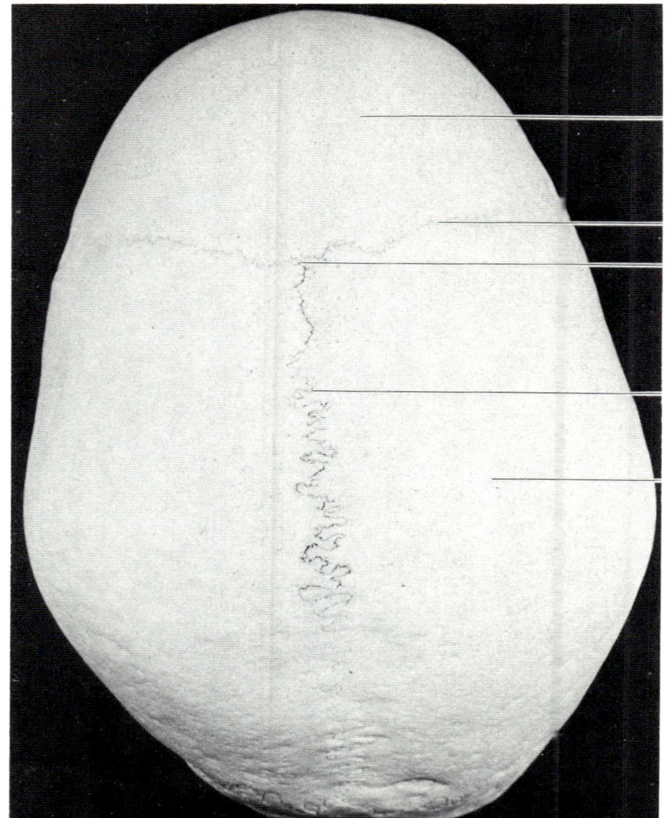

Figure 1-3. Skull—top view

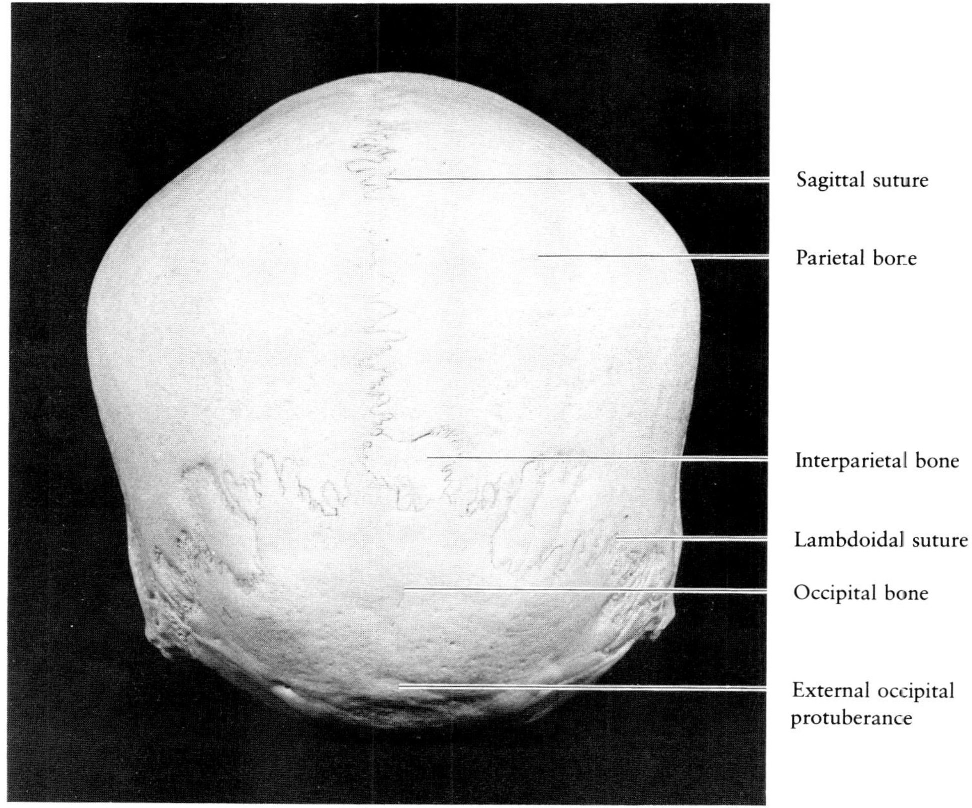

Figure 1-4. Skull—viewed from behind

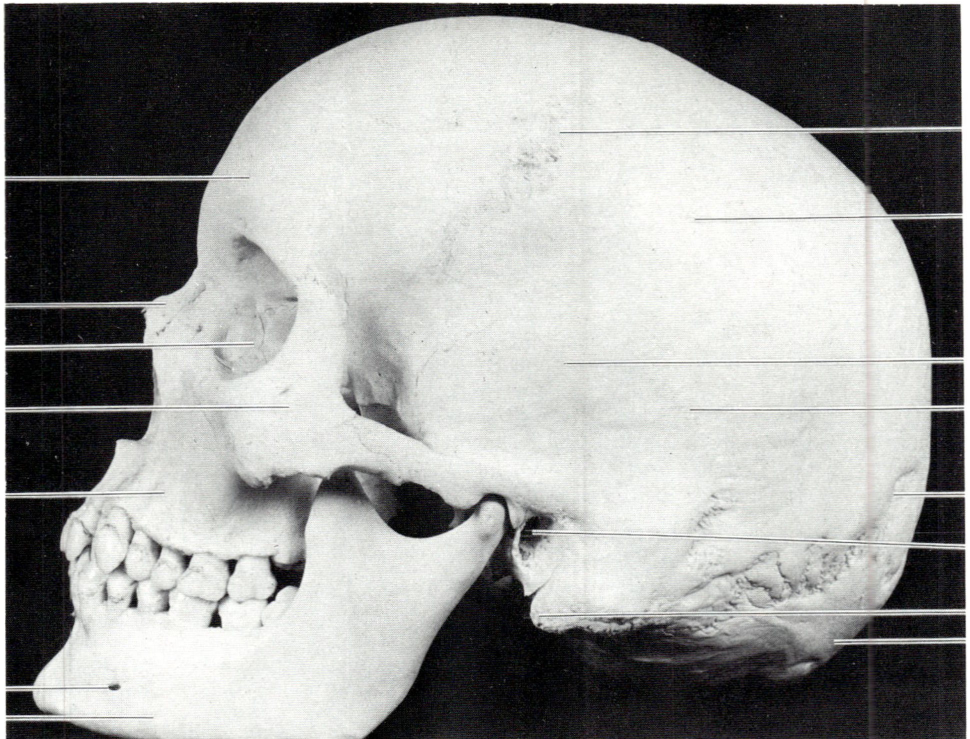

Figure 1-5. Skull—side view

from the tympanic portion of the temporal bone. The squamotympanic fissure separates the two parts.

b. *Tympanic part.* This curved plate forms the anterior, inferior, and posterior walls of the external auditory meatus. It also forms the posterior surface of the mandibular fossa, as noted above.

c. *Styloid part.* This pointed process is about 2.5 cm long and projects downward from the posterior aspect of the tympanic portion. Posterior to this process is the stylomastoid foramen, through which the facial nerve passes.

d. *Petromastoid part.* This part has two divisions: (i) the petrous portion and (ii) the mastoid portion.

i. The *petrous portion* is reputed to be the hardest bone in the body. Pyramidal in form, it projects into the base of the cranial cavity, being lodged between the sphenoid and occipital bones. It houses and protects the delicate mechanisms of hearing and equilibrium.

ii. The *mastoid portion* is located exteriorly on the skull posterior to the external auditory meatus. Its process—the mastoid process—is blunt and rounded and projects downward. The mastoid air cells are located within the mastoid portion of the temporal bone.

Because of its importance in housing the hearing and equilibrium mechanisms, a detailed study of the temporal bone is necessary. Table I lists important landmarks on the temporal bone and their functions. The location of these structures should be learned using Figures 1-6, 1-7, and 1-8, as well as illustrations in other reference texts.

Two bones form the base of the cranium.

5. *Sphenoid.* The sphenoid is a large, complex, butterfly-shaped bone located in front of the occipital and temporal bones. Numerous landmarks are found on this bone, since it forms the major part of the base of the skull. However, only the most pertinent ones will be discussed. Superiorly (inside the cranial cavity) are found the tuberculum sellae and hypophyseal fossa (Figure 1-9). Protruding perpendicularly from the inferior surface are the pterygoid processes (Figure 1-10). These processes divide into medial and lateral pterygoid

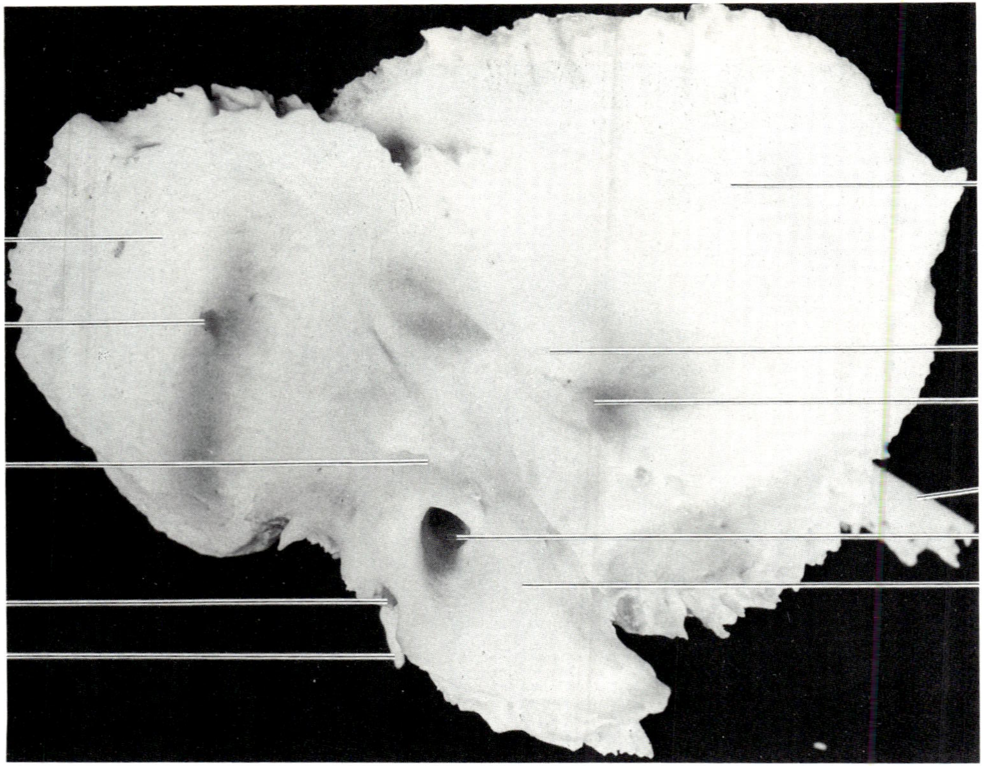

Figure 1-7. Temporal bone—medial aspect

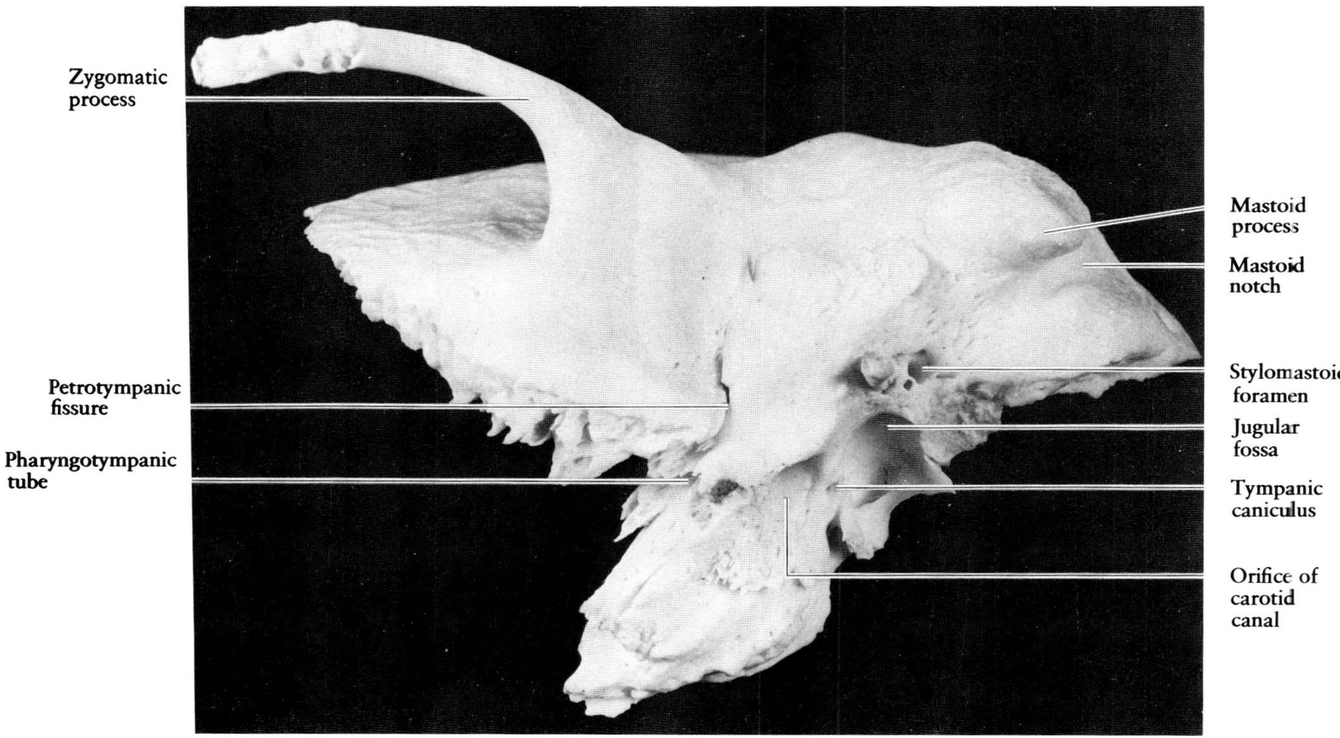

Figure 1-8. Temporal bone—inferior aspect

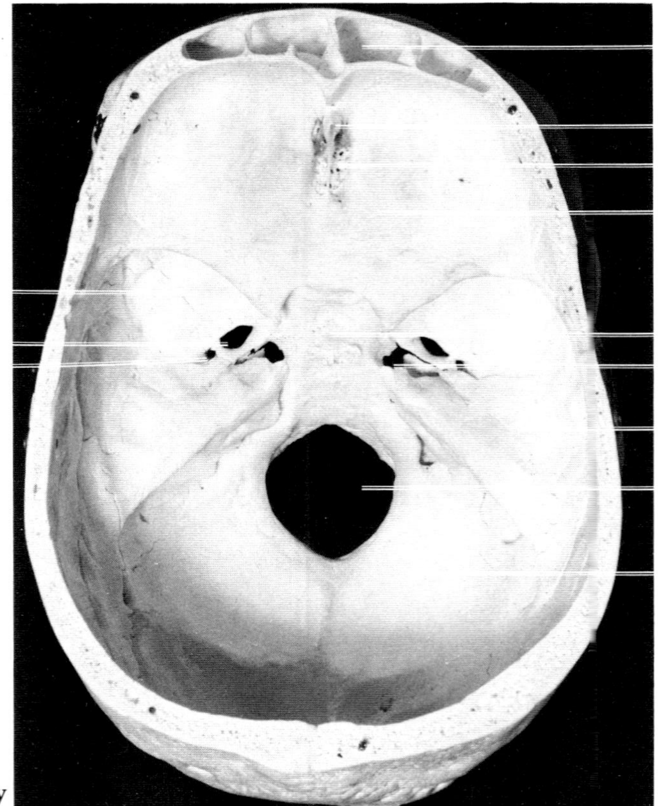

Figure 1-9. Skull—floor of cranial cavity

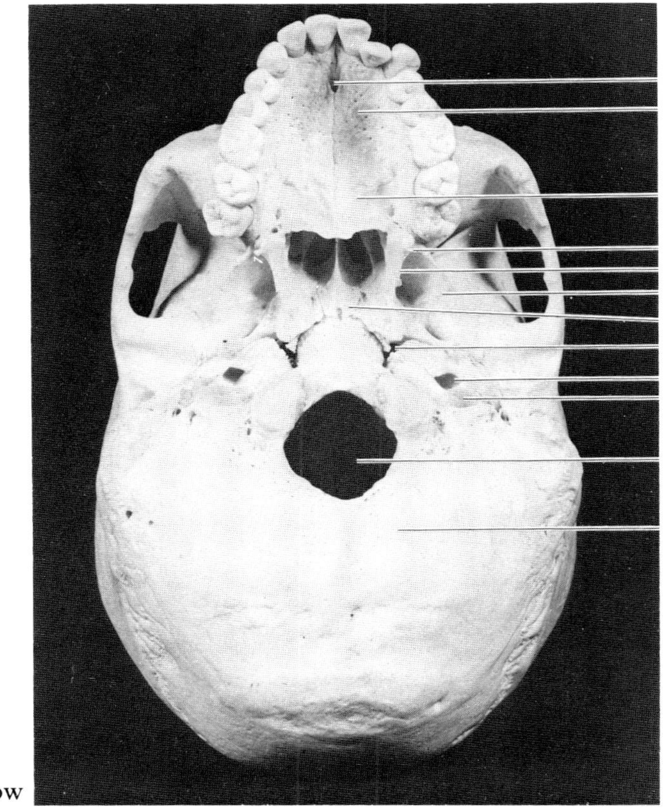

Figure 1-10. Skull—viewed from below

from the roof of the nasal cavity to the brain. Air spaces located lateral to the cribriform plate on both sides form the ethmoidal air sinuses. The midline perpendicular plate of the ethmoid forms the upper part of the nasal septum.

B. Facial bones

There are 14 facial bones that make up the noncranial part of the skull.

1. *Inferior nasal concha* (paired). This is located on the lateral walls of the nasal cavity and overhangs a space called the inferior meatus.
2. *Lacrimal bone* (paired). A small bone located on the medial wall of the orbit. It contains a groove that lodges the nasolacrimal duct.
3. *Vomer.* The vomer is difficult to observe in the intact skull. It forms the inferior part of the nasal septum and articulates superiorly with the perpendicular plate of the ethmoid bone.
4. *Nasal bone* (paired). Lies in the bridge of the nose.
5. *Maxilla* (paired). This complex bone forms the upper jaw and roof of the mouth and consists of a body and four processes.

    a. *Body.* Contains the maxillary air sinus.
    b. *Frontal process.* Extends upward; forms the lateral part of nose and articulates with the frontal, nasal, and ethmoid bones.
    c. *Zygomatic process.* Extends laterally to articulate with the zygomatic bone.
    d. *Alveolar process.* A thick inferior ridge that bears the teeth.
    e. *Palatine process.* Forms the anterior part of the hard palate. The medial parts articulate with each other in the midline and with the vomer. Posteriorly, it articulates with the palatine bone.

6. *Zygomatic bone* (paired). This is the cheek bone, and it consists of a roughly quadrilateral-shaped body and two processes. The frontal process articulates with the frontal bone,

and the temporal process articulates with the temporal bone. The body articulates with the maxilla.

7. *Palatine bone* (paired). This is a small but complex bone that contributes to the floor and lateral walls of the nasal cavity, roof of the mouth, and the floor of the orbit. Its horizontal plate is best seen where it articulates with the palatal processes of the maxilla and forms the posterior part of the hard palate.
8. *Mandible.* This is a horse-shoe shaped bone with a body and two vertical rami. Each ramus is surmounted by a rounded condyloid process and a pointed coronoid process. The head of the condyloid process articulates with the mandibular fossa at the temporomandibular joint. The coronoid process serves as a point of attachment for the temporalis muscle. The vertical posterior border of the ramus meets the lower border of the body (base of the mandible) at the angle of the mandible. The body of the mandible is divided into two parts: (a) The upper or alveolar part, which contains the sockets for the lower teeth, and (b) the lower border or base, which is thick and rounded. There are numerous important landmarks on the mandible, and these are listed in Table II. These structures should be identified using Figure 1-11 and 1-12 and the actual specimen.

Table II. Landmarks of the mandible

Structure	*Function*
Lateral surface (external)	
Mental foramen	Permits exit of the mental nerve and vessels
Mental protuberance	Chin
Mental tubercle	Lateral limit of chin
Incisive fossa	Gives origin to mentalis and part of orbicularis oris muscle
Oblique line	Separates alveolar bone from body of mandible
Medial surface (internal)	
Genial tubercles	Provides attachments for the genioglossus and geniohyoid muscles
Mylohyoid line	Divides internal surface of body into two areas and provides attachment for the mylohyoid muscle
Sublingual fossa	Lodges sublingual salivary gland
Submandibular fossa	Lodges submandibular salivary gland
Digastric fossa	Provides attachment for the anterior belly of digastric muscle
Mandibular foramen	Permits entrance of the inferior alveolar nerve and vessels
Lingula	Provides attachment for the sphenomandibular ligament
Mylohyoid groove	Lodges the mylohyoid nerve and vessels

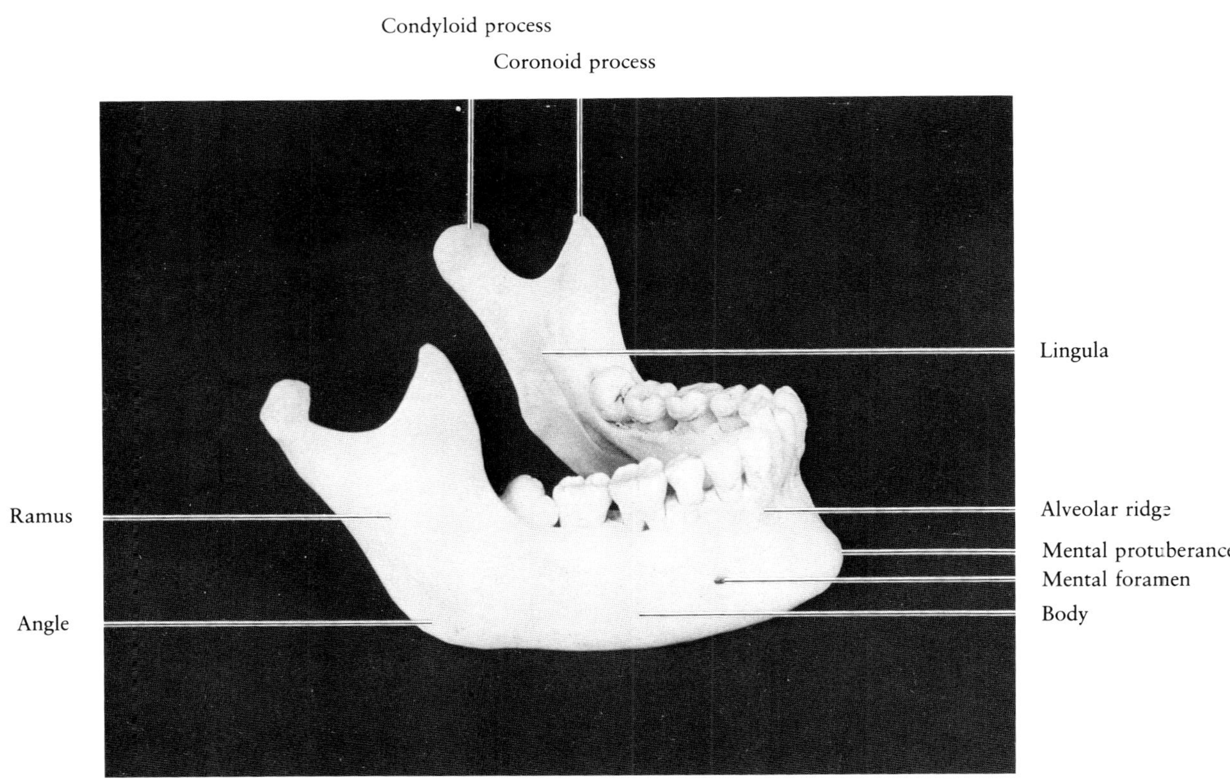

Figure 1-11. Mandible—side view

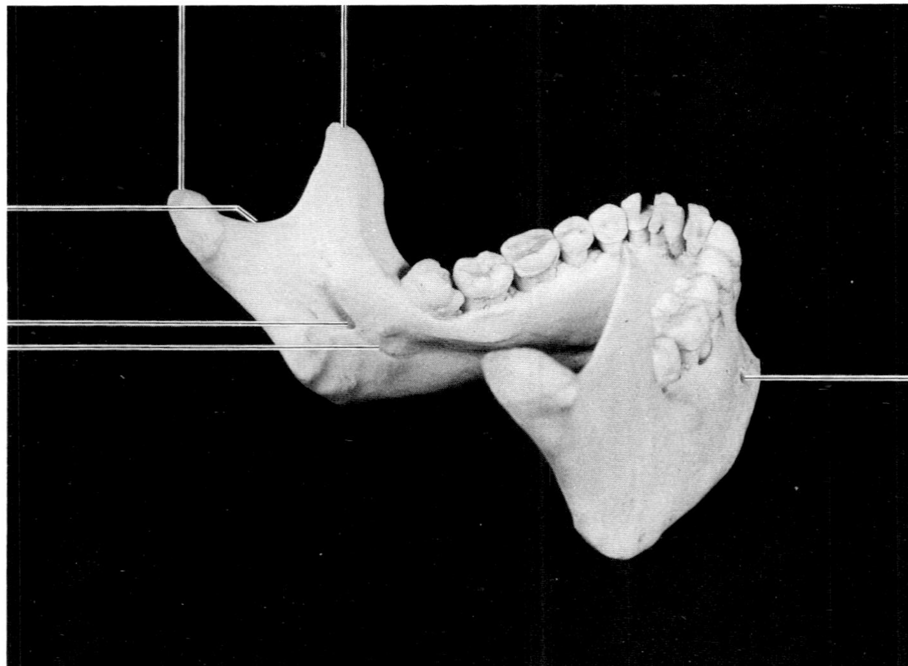

Figure 1-12. Mandible—oblique view

REVIEW QUESTIONS

1. What are the functions of the skeleton?
2. How many bones are there in the skull?
3. Name the three basic types of joints that may be found in the skeleton.
4. Which type of joint permits free movement?
5. Name the eight bones that make up the cranium.
6. Name the parts of the temporal bone.
7. List the major landmarks on the temporal bone, indicating the function of each.
8. Name the 14 bones that make up the facial skeleton.
9. List five landmarks on the lateral surface of the mandible.
10. List eight landmarks on the medial surface of the mandible.

SUGGESTED READINGS

Crouch, J. E. *Functional Human Anatomy,* 3rd ed. Lea & Febiger, Philadelphia, 1978, pp. 83–142.

Hollinshead, W. H. *Textbook of Anatomy,* 3rd ed. Harper & Row, New York, 1974, pp. 788–847.

2
The Hearing Apparatus

Inner Ear

OSSEOUS LABYRINTH

Semicircular Canals

Vestibule

Cochlea

MEMBRANOUS LABYRINTH

Semicircular Ducts

Utricle

Saccule

Cochlear Duct and Organ of Corti

FACIAL NERVE

THE EAR

The term "ear" refers to the structure that contains the vestibulocochlear organs responsible for the senses of equilibrium and hearing. These organs are located within the temporal bone, with the delicate sense organs being encapsulated and protected by the hard petrous portion (Figure 2-1).

The ear may be divided into three parts for descriptive purposes as follows:

1. The external ear, which comprises the auricle (pinna), the external auditory meatus, and the tympanic membrane.
2. The middle ear or tympanic cavity, which contains the auditory ossicles and their associated muscles and tendons. It is in communication with the pharynx and mastoid air cells.

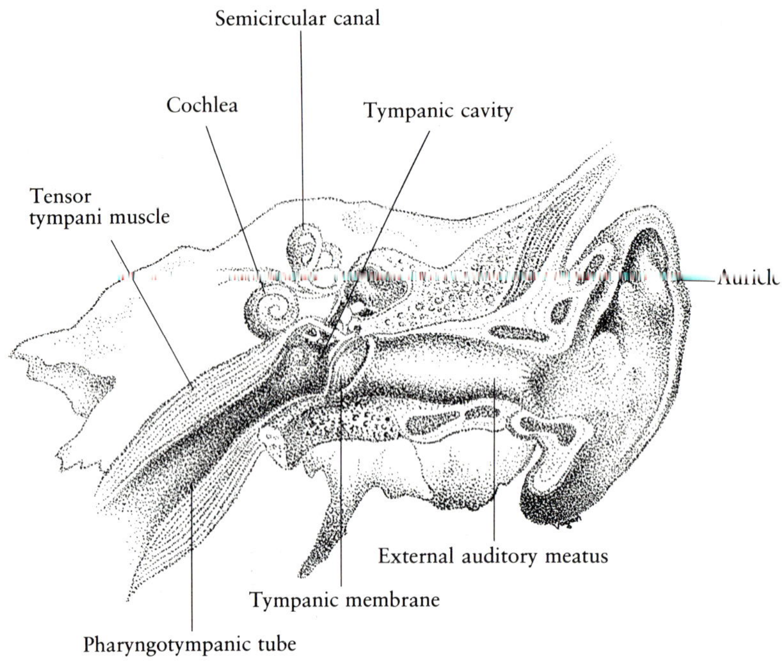

Figure 2-1. The ear

3. The inner ear, which comprises a series of complicated fluid-filled spaces known as the labyrinth.

Each of these sections will be described in detail, and the student is advised to refer to the illustrations frequently while following the written text.

External Ear

The external ear is specialized for the gathering and conduction of sound to the tympanic membrane (eardrum), which separates the external ear from the tympanic cavity.

AURICLE

The *auricle,* or pinna, is a roughly C-shaped flap of tissue attached to the side of the head. It is the most visible part of the hearing mechanism. It is flexible, consisting of a thin, elastic fibrocartilage core covered by skin, and is attached to the surrounding structures of the skull by muscles and ligaments. It is continuous with the cartilaginous part of the external acoustic meatus. The surface of the auricle is uneven and filled with numerous eminences and depressions. Although there is great genetic variation in the size and shape of the auricle, most of the structures are constant. These are shown in Figure 2-2.

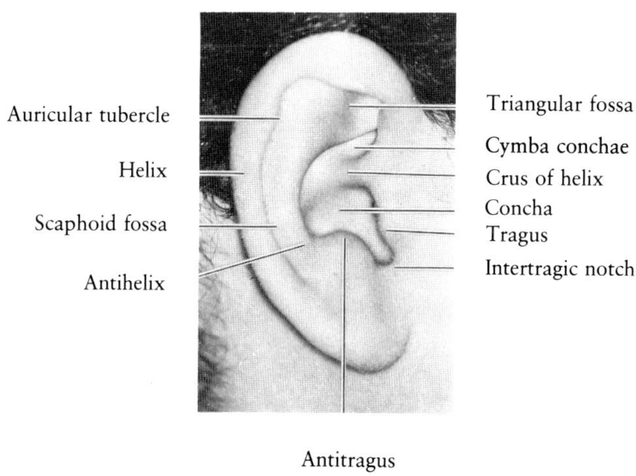

Figure 2-2. Auricle (pinna)

There are extrinsic and intrinsic muscles of the auricle, but these are usually regarded as vestigial, and except in rare cases, no movement of the auricle can be voluntarily elicited. It should be pointed out that lower animals, such as dogs, cats, and horses, retain the capacity to control the position of the auricle voluntarily.

There are three sources of blood supply to the auricle.

1. Posterior auricular branch of the external carotid artery
2. Anterior auricular branch of the superficial temporal artery
3. A branch of the occipital artery

Accompanying veins subsequently drain the organ into the external jugular vein.

The lymphatics empty into the parotid, upper deep cervical, and mastoid lymph nodes. The sensory innervation of the auricle is accomplished via five nerves. These are the great auricular nerve, the lesser occipital nerve, the auricular branch of the vagus, the auriculotemporal nerve, and the facial nerve. It is interesting to note that the auricle contains many acupuncture points.

EXTERNAL AUDITORY MEATUS

The *external auditory meatus* is an oval canal, approximately 2.5 cm in length, that extends from the bottom of the concha of the auricle to the tympanic membrane (Figure 2-1). Its path is roughly S shaped, with the lateral portion of the canal being directed medially forward and upward and the medial portion directed forward and downward. It consists of two parts. The lateral one third is cartilaginous and continuous with the auricle. It is attached by fibrous tissue to the bony medial two thirds, the cavity in the petrous portions of the temporal bone. The diameter of the bony canal is slightly less than that of the cartilaginous portion, and its medial end is sloped such that its anterior wall projects about 4 mm beyond its posterior wall. This end is marked by a narrow groove, called the tympanic sulcus, to which the tympanic membrane is attached.

The skin covering the auricle continues into and lines the external auditory meatus and the tympanic membrane. It is thin skin that is closely attached to the underlying cartilage and bone of the canal. Hair follicles and sebaceous and ceruminous glands are found in the skin covering the membranous part of the canal. These structures perform a protective function. Cerumen (ear wax) is formed from the glandular secretions and entrapped particles of dust.

Blood is supplied to the canal via the posterior auricular branch of the external carotid artery, the deep auricular branch of the maxillary, and the auricular branches of the superficial temporal artery. Venous drainage is by way of the external jugular and maxillary veins as well as the pterygoid plexus. The lymphatics drain with those of the auricle.

The auriculotemporal branch of the mandibular nerve supplies the anterior and upper walls of the meatus, and the posterior and inferior walls are supplied by the auricular branch of the vagus.

TYMPANIC MEMBRANE

The *tympanic membrane* is a thin oval structure, about 10 mm in its longer diamter, and lies at the end of the external auditory meatus, separating the external ear from the tympanic cavity. Because of the difference in length between the roof and the floor of the end of the external acoustic meatus, the tympanic membrane occupies an oblique position. The angle formed by the tympanic membrane and the floor of the meatus is about 55°.

When examined with reflected light, the membrane has a glistening pearly gray appearance. It is semitransparent, and the outline of the handle of the malleus, which is attached to its medial surface, may be seen extending upward and forward. The center of the membrane is slightly concave and is called the umbo. Because of the concavity and the oblique attitude of the membrane, its anterior inferior quadrant glows brightly, and this is known as the cone of light (Figure 2-3).

The margin of the circumference of the membrane is thickened and forms a fibrocartilaginous ring that is attached to the tympanic sulcus of the bony part of the external acoustic meatus. This sulcus is deficient superiorly, and from the ends of the notch, two folds of the membrane, known as the anterior and posterior malleolar folds, are seen. These folds are inserted on the lateral process of the malleus. The small flap of the tympanic membrane located above these folds is called the pars flaccida of the tympanic membrane. The major part of the membrane is taut and is affixed to the tympanic sulcus. It is known as the pars tensa.

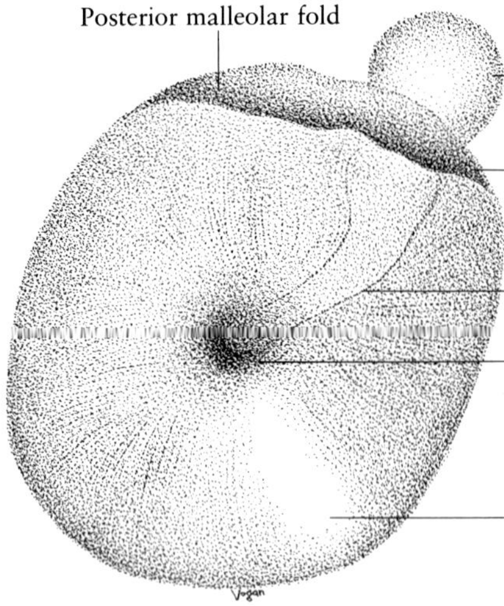

Figure 2-3. Tympanic membrane

Structure. The tympanic membrane is a three-layered membrane. The lateral surface is derived from the skin that lines the external acoustic meatus. The intermediate layer is fibrous connective tissue, and the medial layer is continuous with the mucosa of the tympanic cavity. The arterial supply of the tympanic membrane is derived from the deep auricular and stylomastoid branches of the maxillary artery. The superficial veins empty into the external jugular vein. The deep veins drain either into the transverse sinus and veins of the dura or into the plexus of veins on the auditory tube. The nerve supply is from the auriculotemporal branch of the mandibular nerve, auricular branch of the vagus nerve, and the tympanic branch of the glossopharyngeal nerve.

Middle Ear

TYMPANIC CAVITY

The *tympanic cavity* is an air space within the temporal bone. It is lined by a mucous membrane and contains the auditory ossicles (malleus, incus, and stapes) that transmit sound from the tympanic membrane to the inner ear mechanism (Figure 2-1). The tympanic cavity also communicates with the nasopharynx by way of the pharyngotympanic (auditory or eustachian) tube and with the mastoid anthrum and air cells. The cavity may be divided into two parts: 1. the tympanic cavity proper, which lies opposite the tympanic membrane, and 2. the epitympanic recess (attic), which is the part of the cavity above the membrane. The epitympanic recess contains the head of the malleus and most of the incus. It should be noted that the tympanic cavity is a very small cavity. Its greatest measurements are 15 mm each for the vertical and anteroposterior diameters. The transverse diameter is largest (about 6 mm) above and only about 2 mm opposite the center of the tympanic membrane. The cavity may be thought of as a cube with a floor, roof, and anterior, posterior, lateral, and medial walls (Figure 2-4). To help visualize the relationships, imagine yourself standing in the tympanic cavity of the right ear. You are standing on the floor. If you look up, you will see the roof. Straight ahead is the anterior wall and behind you is the posterior wall. To your right is the tympanic membrane (lateral

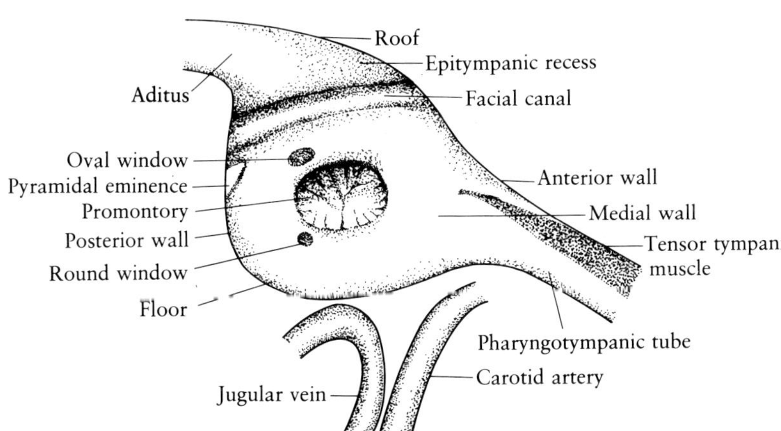

Figure 2-4. Schematic diagram of tympanic cavity

wall) and to your left is the medial wall. We will now discuss the structures located on each wall.

Floor. The floor consists of a thin plate of bone that overlies the jugular fossa (seen when the temporal bone was studied earlier). In the floor near the medial wall is a small aperture through which the tympanic branch of the glossopharyngeal nerve passes.

Roof. The roof also consists of a thin plate of bone called the tegmen tympani. It forms part of the floor of the cranial cavity.

Anterior Wall. Because the roof and the floor slope toward each other, the anterior wall is relatively small. The upper part consists of the openings of two canals placed one upon each other, and the lower part is the upward-sloping floor. The upper of the two canals lodges the tensor tympani muscle and is separated from the lower bony part of the pharyngotympanic tube by a thin bony septum. The lower part of the anterior wall forms the posterior wall of the carotid canal. Perforations for the passage of the chorda tympani nerve, the superior and inferior corticotympanic nerves, and the tympanic branch of the internal carotid artery are present.

Posterior Wall. The posterior wall is an incomplete wall. Its lower part is bony, but its upper part consists of an opening known as the aditus (aditus ad antrum), which connects the tympanic cavity with the mastoid antrum and mastoid air cells. The mastoid air cells are a series of communicating, mucosa-lined air-filled spaces located within the mastoid process of the temporal bone. Three other structures are located on the posterior wall.

1. The *fossa incudis* is a small depression in the lower and posterior part of the epitympanic recess. The short process of the incus is attached to the fossa incudis by ligamentous fibers.

2. The *pyramidal eminence* is a short, hollow, conical projection located at the junction of the posterior and medial wall close to the fenestra vestibuli. It contains the stapedius muscle.

3. The *posterior canaliculus* of the chorda, located near the posterior edge of the tympanic membrane close to its top, permits the entrance of the chorda tympani nerve into the tympanic cavity.

Lateral Wall. The lateral wall is composed of the tympanic membrane with the attached handle of the malleus as previously described. The chorda tympani nerve crosses the upper part of the tympanic membrane from the posterior wall to its exit on the anterior wall.

Medial Wall. The medial wall is perhaps the most important wall of the tympanic cavity. It is also the lateral surface of the internal ear. Several structures important to the hearing mechanism are located on this wall.

1. A prominent bulge, called the *promontory,* is usually the most visible structure. It is formed by the basal turn of the cochlea of the internal ear. Its surface is furrowed and lodges the nerves of the tympanic plexus (from tympanic branch of ninth cranial nerve).
2. The *fenestra vestibuli,* or oval window, is located above and behind the promontory. It leads into the vestibule of the inner ear. This window is closed by the base of the stapes, the circumference of which is attached to the margin of the window by the annular ligament.
3. The *fenestra cochleae,* or round window, is located below and behind the promontory. It leads into the scala tympani of the cochlea and is closed by the secondary tympanic membrane.
4. The prominent ridge located above the fenestra vestibuli is called the *prominence of the facial canal.* This ridge marks the path of the facial nerve as it runs backward on the medial wall and then descends behind the posterior wall to the stylomastoid foramen.
5. The *processus cochleariformis* is a thin, curled ledge of bone continuous with the septum that separates the canal for the tensor tympani muscle from the bony part of the pharyngotympanic tube. It projects almost to the upper margin of the fenestra vestibuli, and its posterior end is turned like a pulley. The tendon of the tensor tympani muscle lies on this shelf of bone and plays over the pulley as it turns to insert onto the handle of the malleus.

6. A final landmark is the *sinus tympani.* This is a small depression behind the promontory and marks the location of the ampulla of the posterior semicircular canal.

The major structures located within the middle ear or tympanic cavity are the ossicles of the middle ear and two small muscles—the tensor tympani and stapedius muscles. It should also be remembered that the chorda tympani nerve passes through the tympanic cavity.

OSSICLES

The *ossicles* are a chain of the three movable bones that extend from the tympanic membrane to the fenestra vestibuli. They serve to transmit sound vibrations from the tympanic membrane to the inner ear. The names of the bones are the malleus, incus, and stapes (Figure 2-5). The malleus is attached to the tympanic membrane, and the stapes is attached to the fenestra vestibuli. The incus is placed between the two and articulates with both. The articulations are synovial joints.

Malleus. The *malleus* is the largest of the ossicles and is shaped somewhat like a hammer. It is 8 to 9 mm long and consists of a head, neck, and three processes—the anterior process, the lateral process, and the manubrium, or handle. The head is the largest part of the bone and projects up into the epitympanic recess. It articulates posteriorly with the incus. The head is attached to the roof by superior mallear ligaments.

The narrow part below the head is known as the neck. The short anterior process and larger lateral process is located just below the neck. The anterior process is connected by the anterior mallear ligaments to the petrotympanic fissure. The lateral process serves as a point of attachment for the malleolar folds.

The manubrium extends downward medially and backward and is embedded in the center of the tympanic membrane. The tendon of the tensor tympani muscle is attached to a slight projection of the upper part of its medial surface.

Incus. The *incus* is shaped somewhat like a molar tooth. It consists of a body and two diverging arms. The body lies in the epitympanic recess and articulates with the head of the malleus.

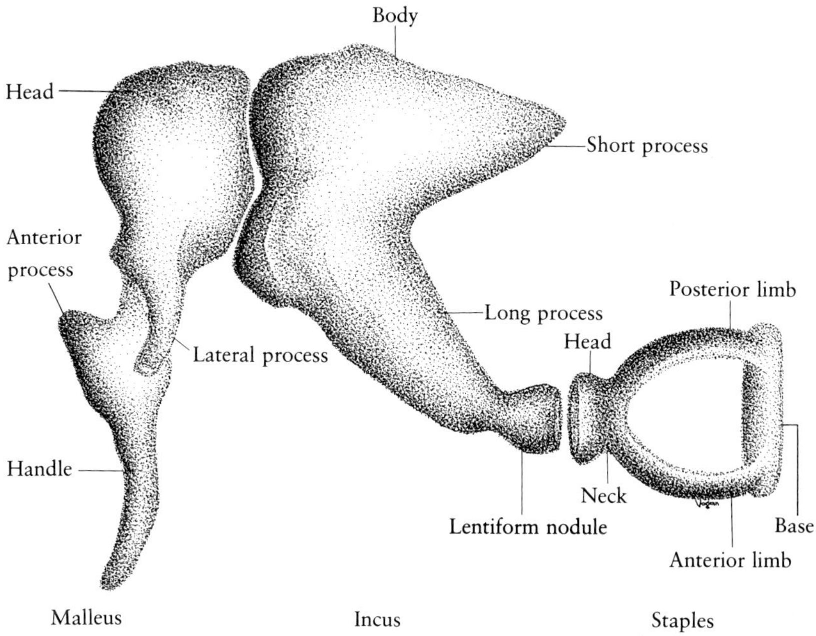

Figure 2-5. Ossicles of the ear

The short crus (process) lies in the fossa incudis, to which it is attached by ligamentous fibers. The long crus (process) extends downward and turns medially to end in the knoblike lentiform nodule, which articulates with the head of the stapes.

Stapes. The *stapes,* a stirrup-shaped bone, consists of a head, neck, two limbs, and a base. The head is directed laterally and articulates with the lentiform nodule (above). The stapedius muscle is inserted into the neck. The base of the stapes is attached to the fenestra vestibuli (oval window) by a annular ligament.

MUSCLES

The *tensor tympani muscle* originates from the cartilage of the pharyngotympanic tube and adjoining greater wing of the sphenoid. It passed through the upper bony canal in the anterior wall of the tympanic cavity. Its tendon rests on the cochleariform process and turns laterally round the pulley-shaped end to insert on the upper end of the handle of the malleus (Figure 2-1). This muscle is innervated by a branch of the mandibular nerve. Its action is to tense the tympanic membrane by drawing the handle of the malleus medially.

The *stapedius muscle* arises from the interior walls of the pyramidal eminence on the posterior wall of the tympanic cavity. Its tendon emerges from the apex of the pyramid (see Figure 2-10) and is inserted into the posterior surface of the neck of the stapes. This muscle is innervated by a small twig from the facial nerve. Its action is to prevent excessive oscillations of the stapes.

PHARYNGOTYMPANIC TUBE (EUSTACHIAN OR AUDITORY TUBE)

The pharyngotympanic tube provides for communication of the middle ear cavity with the nasopharynx and permits the equalization of pressure on both sides of the tympanic membrane. It may also serve as a passage for the transfer of bacterial or other infection from the pharynx to the tympanic cavity.

The tube is trumpet shaped, about 25 mm long, extending from the anterior wall of the tympanic cavity to the lateral wall of the nasopharynx, and consists of two parts—a bony part and a cartilaginous part.

Bony Part. The bony part is located in temporal bone and runs from the anterior wall of the tympanic cavity to an opening on the base of skull behind and medial to the spine of the sphenoid.

Cartilaginous Part. This triangular cartilaginous plate is curled to form the upper, lower, and medial wall of the tube. The lateral wall is filled in by fibrous tissue. The apex of the tube is attached to the bony part, but the base is curved and free, opening into the lateral wall of the nasopharynx, where attachments of the tensor veli palatini muscle causes the tube to open during yawning and swallowing.

The entire pharyngotympanic tube is lined by a mucosa that is thin in the osseous part. It is thicker in the cartilaginous part, and mucous glands and lymphoid tissue are present. Nerves from the tympanic plexus and the pharyngeal branch of the sphenopalatine ganglion supply the pharyngotympanic tube.

The Inner Ear

The inner ear is enclosed within the petrous portion of the temporal bone and contains the organs of equilibrium and hearing. These organs are anatomically linked and are supplied by branches of the vestibulocochlear or eighth cranial nerve. Structurally, the inner ear consists of two sets of fluid-filled cavities: the osseous labyrinth and the membranous labyrinth. The membranous labyrinth, which contains the delicate sensory organs, is completely enclosed and protected by the osseous labyrinth.

OSSEOUS LABYRINTH

The *osseous labyrinth* consists of a series of continuous spaces (perilymphatic spaces) surrounded by bone (otic capsule). The perilymphatic space is crossed by small, delicate trabeculae and lined by endosteum. The fluid found in this space is called perilymph. Three major parts of the osseous labyrinth are recognized. These are the semicircular canals, the vestibule, and the cochlea (Figure 2-6).

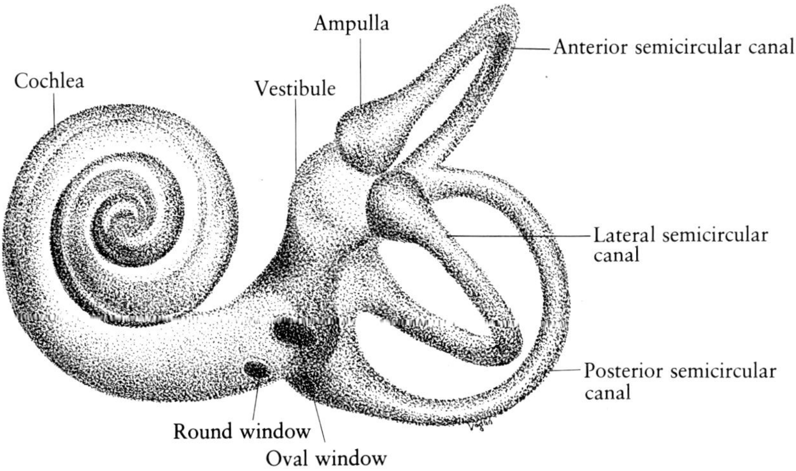

Figure 2-6. Osseous labyrinth

Semicircular Canals. The *semicircular canals,* of which there are three, are located above and behind the vestibule, The anterior and posterior semicircular canals are located in the vertical plane at right angles to each other, and the lateral semicircular canal assumes the horizontal plane when the head is flexed 30°. Each canal forms approximately two thirds of a circle and is ampullated at one end. The anterior and posterior canals share a common arm, the crus commune, which opens into the medial part of the vestibule. The semicircular canals enclose the semicircular ducts, which will be described later.

Vestibule. The *vestibule* is the middle dilated portion of the osseous labyrinth. It communicates with the cochlea anteriorly and with the semicircular canals posteriorly. It is closely applied to the medial wall of the tympanic cavity such that the fenestra vestibuli and fenestra cochleae located on the vestibule were previously identified as structures located on the medial wall of the tympanic cavity. A small canal, called the aqueduct of the vestibule, passes posteroinferiorly to open on the posterior surface of the petrous bone. It transmits the endolymphatic duct and sac. The vestibule houses the utricle and saccule in elliptical and spherical recesses. These will be described with the membranous labyrinth.

Cochlea. The *cochlea* somewhat resembles the shell of a snail. It is a helical tube of approximately two and three-fourths turns (Figure 2-7). The wide basal turn forms the promontory of the medial wall of the tympanic cavity. The apex is pointed and directed anterolaterally.

The center of the cochlea consists of a bony core called the modiolus, which transmits the cochlear nerve and spiral ganglia. Projecting laterally from the modiolus is the osseous spiral lamina, which partially divides the cochlea into two portions, the scala vestibuli anteriorly and the scala tympani posteriorly. At the apex of the cochlea, these two chambers are in communication with each other at the helicotrema. The division of the cochlea is completed by the cochlear duct. To assist in understanding the relationships, visualize a common screw as the modiolus, with the flanges of the screw being the osseous spiral lamina. Next visualize a piece of rubber hose wrapped around the screw

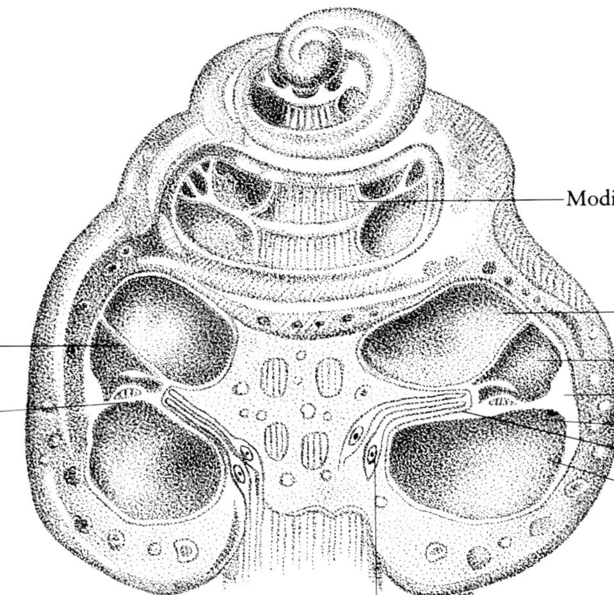

Figure 2-7. Cochlea

in such a way that the flanges of the screw sink into the hose and partially divide it into two chambers. The division of the chambers is completed by the presence of the cochlear duct attached to the edge of the osseous spiral lamina.

The scale vestibuli begins at the fenestra vestibuli, which is occupied by the base of the stapes. The scala tympani ends at the fenestra cochleae (round window), which is closed by the secondary tympanic membrane. Both scalae are filled with perilymph. The cochlear canaliculus runs from the lower end of the scala tympani near the fenestra cochlea to the anterior margin of the jugular foramen. It transmits the microscopic perilymphatic duct (or aqueduct of the cochlea), which opens into the subarachnoid space of the posterior cranial fossa. As a result, the perilymphatic channels are in communication with the subarachnoid space, and perilymph is similar in composition to cerebrospinal fluid.

MEMBRANOUS LABYRINTH

The *membranous labyrinth* comprises a series of connected ducts and tubes completely housed within the osseous labyrinth. It consists of the semicircular ducts, utricle, and saccule, and cochlear duct (Figure 2-8). These tubes and ducts are filled with endolymph and are surrounded by the perilymph of the osseous labyrinth. Endolymph is a relatively viscous fluid that is produced by the stria vascularis of the cochlear duct (Figure 2-9). It is similar in composition to intracellular fluid. Absorption of endolympth occurs through the endolymphatic sac into the surrounding venules in the base of the brain.

Semicircular Ducts. The *semicircular ducts* lie within the semicircular canals and are about one fourth the diameter of the canal. Each duct has an ampullated end that contains the ampullary crest. The ampullary crest consists of neuroepithelial cells, the hair of which projects into a gelatinous mass called the cupula. Movement of the endolymph apparently distorts the cupula and stimulates the hair cells. The semicircular ducts open into the utricle through five openings.

Utricle. The *utricle* is an oval sac that lies in the posterior part of the vestibule. It receives the openings of the semicircular ducts and contains the sense organ called the macula, one of which is

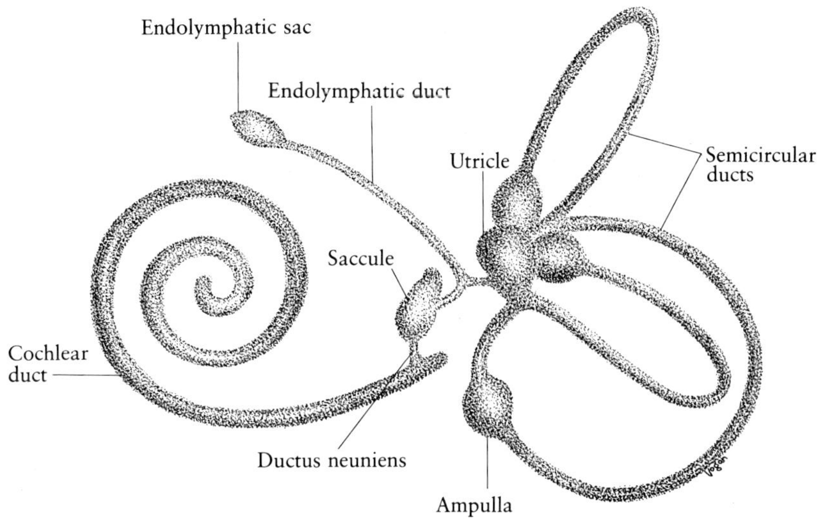

Figure 2-8. Membranous labyrinth

also found in the saccule. The macula consists of neuroepithelial hair cells. The processes from the cells are embedded in a membrane in which are also embedded calcium carbonate crystals called statoconia (otoliths). The maculae are thought to be entirely concerned with balance, and the movement of the statoconia stimulates the neuroepithelial cells which are innervated by fibers of the vestibular division of the eighth cranial nerve.

Anteriorly the utricle is in communication with the saccule through the utriculosaccular duct. The endolymphatic duct leading to the subdural endolymphatic sac is attached to the utriculosaccular duct.

Saccule. The *saccule* is a small round sac located in the anteroinferior part of the vestibule. It contains a macula similar in structure and function to that found in the utricle. In addition to being in communication with the utricle, the saccule is in communication anteriorly with the cochlear duct through the ductus reuniens.

Cochlear Duct and Organ of Corti. The spiral tube comprising

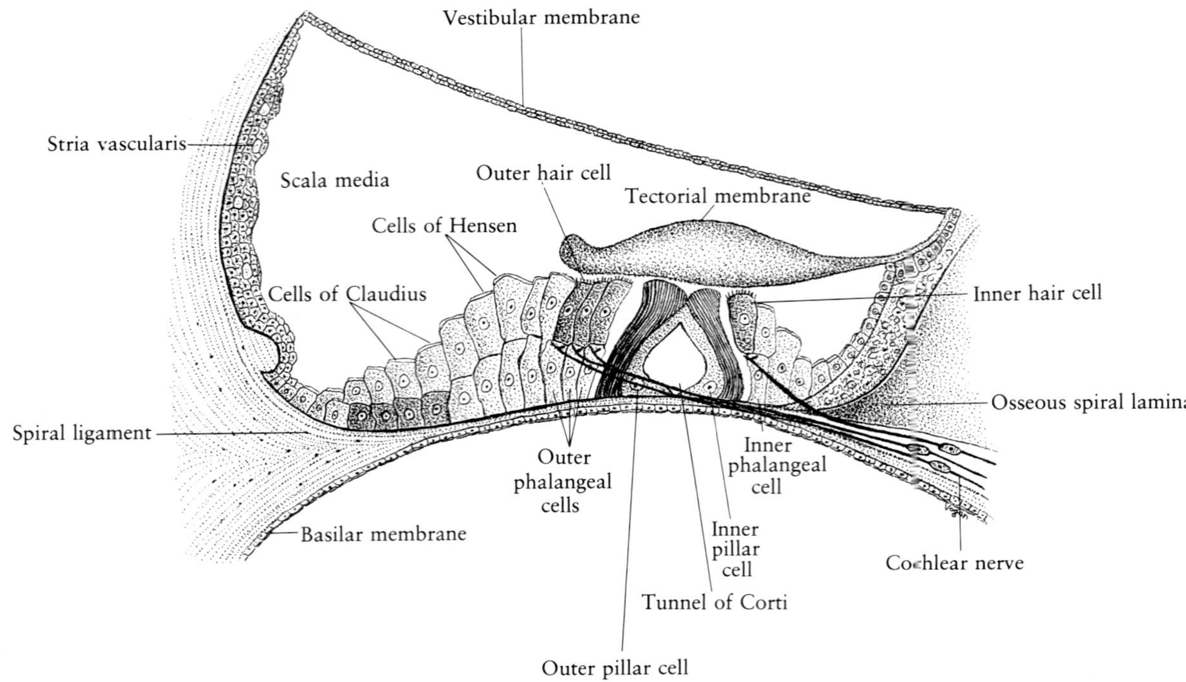

Figure 2-9. Spiral organ of Corti

the cochlear duct and organ of Corti is located within the cochlea. It occupies the lateral portion of the cochlea and completes the division of the cochlea into scala tympani and scala vestibuli (Figure 2-7). Like the rest of the membranous labyrinth, the cochlear duct is filled with endolymph.

Structurally, the cochlear duct (scala media) is somewhat triangular in shape. It has a basilar membrane that extends from the osseous spiral lamina to the spiral ligament.

The basilar membrane supports the hearing organ (organ of Corti) and separates the cochlear duct from the scala tympani. The roof of the cochlear duct is the thin epithelial-covered vestibular membrane that separates it from the scale vestibuli. The third side of the triangle is made up of the spiral ligament, which is actually the thickened periosteal lining of the cochlea.

The sensory mechanism of hearing is known as the organ of Corti. A diagram of a histological section of this organ is shown in Figure 2-9. This cellular structure is maintained along the entire length of the cochlear duct. Many of the cells serve a supportive function, with the hair cells being the sensory cells. An abbreviated description of the functionally more important structures follows.

There are two basic types of supporting cells, the pillar cells and the phalangeal cells. The inner and outer pillar cells are modified phalangeal cells and contain bundles of tonofibrils. These pillar cells enclose the tunnel of Corti. The phalangeal cells are tall, columnar cells found on either side of the tunnel of Corti and serve as support for the sensory hair cells. Usually, there is a single row of inner phalangeal cells and three to five rows of outer phalangeal cells. Correspondingly, there is also only one row of inner hair cells and three to five rows of outer hair cells. These hair cells are characterized by the presence of hairs (actually modified microvilli) that project from their apex and are embedded in the gelatinous tectorial membrane. Dendrites from the cell bodies of the cochlear nerve (cochlear branch of the vestibulocochlear nerve) located in the spiral ganglia terminate on the hair cells. It is not absolutely clear how nerve impulses are initiated in the cochlear nerve as a result of vibration of the perilymph and endolymph. However, it is generally accepted that deflection of the basilar or tectorial membranes causes a "bending" of the sensory hairs, thereby causing the generation of a nerve impulse. Low tones cause vibration of the basilar membrane in the apex of the cochlea, where the membrane is widest. High notes cause a response of the basilar membrane in the basal turn where the membrane is narrowest. The mechanism responsible for regulating this local referral of tones to a particular segment of the basilar membrane is unknown.

FACIAL NERVE

Because of its proximity to the tympanic cavity, the course of the facial nerve in this region will now be discussed. The facial nerve enters the petrous portion of the temporal bone through the internal auditory meatus adjacent to the vestibulocochlear nerve (Figure 2-10). At this point, it consists of two roots that lie above the eighth nerve. The larger of the two roots is the motor root and the other is sensory. These roots fuse within the internal acoustic canal and give rise to the geniculate ganglion, which is located between the upper part of the bony vestibule and the cochlea. The greater superficial petrosal nerve arises from the geniculate ganglion and runs forward to enter the middle cranial fossa of the skull through the slitlike hiatus of the canal of the greater petrosal nerve. The lesser superficial petrosal nerve also arises in part from the geniculate ganglion. One root arises from this ganglion and another from the tympanic plexus of nerves on the promontory of the middle ear (filaments of the tympanic branch of the glossopharyngeal nerve). The two roots fuse and also run forward to enter the middle cranial fossa by a small slit below that of the greater petrosal nerve.

At the geniculate ganglion the facial nerve then turns backward, running in the facial canal previously identified on the medial wall of the tympanic cavity above the promontory. Behind the posterior wall of the tympanic cavity the facial nerve turns abruptly downward to leave the temporal bone at the stylomastoid foramen just below and posterior to the external auditory meatus. In its downward course, before leaving the temporal bone, the facial nerve gives off two important branches.

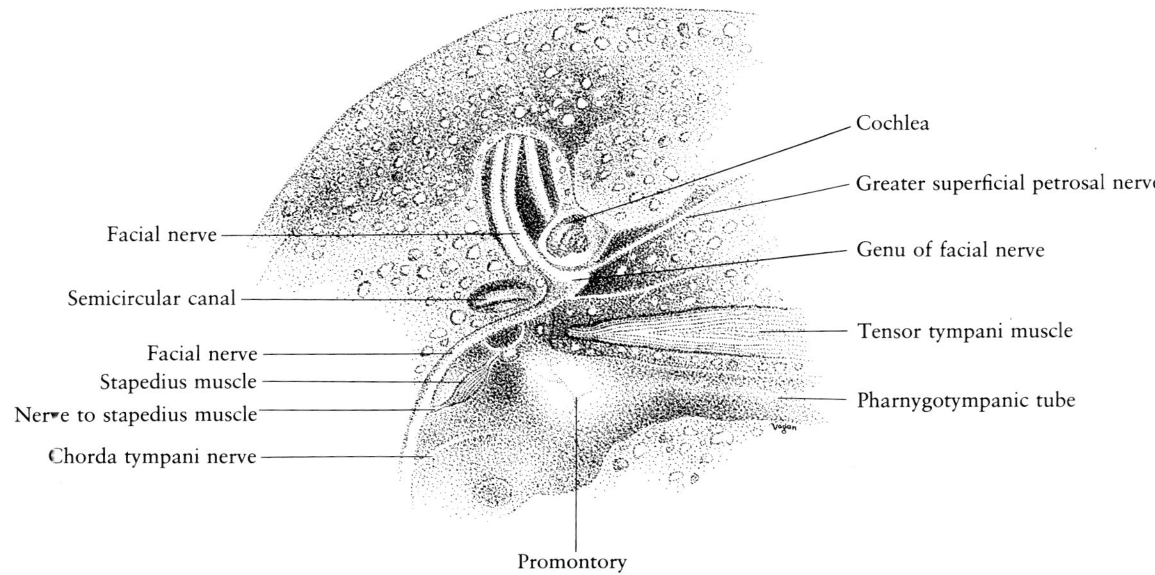

Figure 2-10. Course of facial nerve through temporal bone

1. The nerve to the stapedius muscle, which is a small twig within the bone of the posterior wall of the tympanic cavity.
2. The chorda tympani nerve, which crosses the tympanic membrane from the posterior to the anterior wall of the tympanic cavity. It leaves the tympanic cavity in the exit for the chorda tympani nerve (previously identified), passes through the petrotympanic fissure, and later joins the lingual nerve to the tongue.

REVIEW QUESTIONS

1. Name the three major divisions of the ear.
2. Describe the auricle (pinna) of the ear.
3. What is the role of the middle ear in the function of hearing?
4. List the structures located on the medial wall of the tympanic cavity.
5. With what other chambers of the head is the middle ear in communication and how?
6. Name the ossicles of the middle ear.
7. Name the muscles associated with the tympanic cavity and give their innervation.
8. Describe the parts of the membranous labyrinth of the middle ear and its relationship to the osseous labyrinth.
9. What are the two major branches of the eighth cranial nerve?
10. What is the organ of Corti?
11. Trace the path of the facial nerve through the temporal bone.

SUGGESTED READINGS

Davis, D.V. *Gray's Anatomy,* 34th ed. Longmans, Green & Co. Ltd., London, 1967, pp. 1311–1342.

Ham, A.W. *Histology,* 6th ed. J.B. Lippincott Co. Philadelphia, 1969, pp. 1003–1019.

Zemlin, W.R. *Speech and Hearing Science.* Prentice Hall, Englewood Cliffs, N.J., 1968, pp. 363–416.

3

The Breathing Mechanism

BONY THORAX

Thoracic vertebrae
Ribs
Sternum
Articulations

THORACIC MUSCLES

Intrinsic Muscles of the Thorax

EXTERNAL INTERCOSTALS
INTERNAL INTERCOSTALS
INNERMOST INTERCOSTALS
SUBCOSTALS
TRANSVERSE THORACIC MUSCLES

THE DIAPHRAGM

Sternal Portion
Costal Portion
Lumbar Portion
Crura

RESPIRATORY PASSAGES

Trachea
Bronchi
Lungs

BONY THORAX

The bony thorax is cone shaped and made up of the bodies of the 12 thoracic vertebrae, the 12 pairs of ribs, and the sternum. A brief description of each of these structures follows. For a more comprehensive treatment, the student is referred to any good anatomy text.

Thoracic Vertebrae

There are 12 thoracic vertebrae, and they are basically similar to the other members of the vertebral column (see Figure 3-1). Two important structures located on the thoracic vertebrae are not found on the others, however. Since these vertebrae articulate with the ribs, articular facets (or foveas) are found on the transverse process and on the posterior part of the body. The head of each rib articulates with the superior facet of the body of the thoracic vertebra of the same number and with the inferior facet of the vertebra above. The tubercle of the rib articulates with the transverse process of the vertebra of the corresponding number. An exception is that the transverse process of the eleventh and twelfth vertebrae do not articulate with the ribs. These articulations, where present, are synovial joints, although movement is somewhat restricted.

Ribs

There are usually 12 pairs of ribs. Pairs 1 to 7 are said to be true ribs, since they articulate directly with the sternum by way of individual costal cartilages. Pairs 8 to 12 are called false ribs, since they articulate indirectly with the sternum. The costal cartilage of pairs 8 to 10 joins the costal cartilage of pair 7. Pairs 11 and 12 are embedded in the musculature of the back and are not in direct articulation with the sternum. These are called floating ribs. The parts of a rib are shown in Figure 3-1.

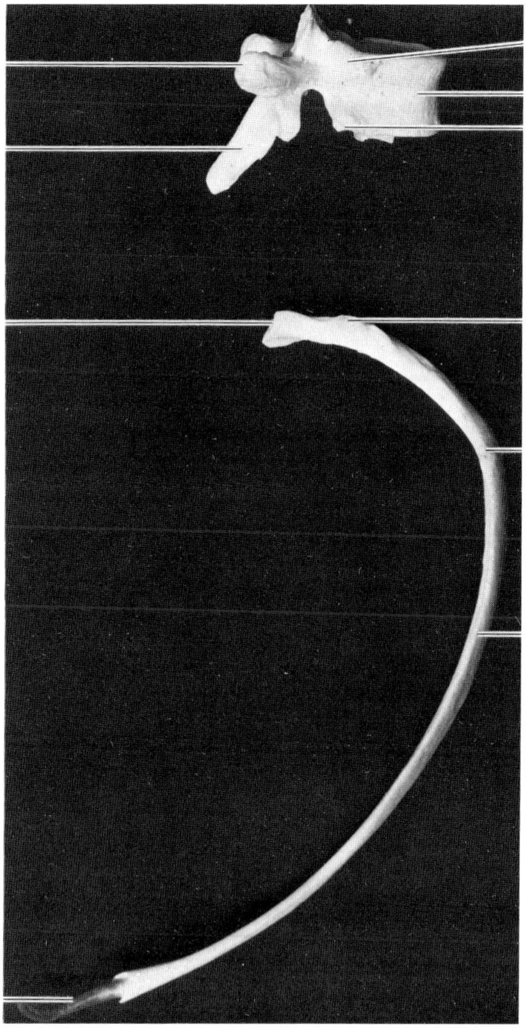

Figure 3-1. Thoracic vertebra and rib

Sternum

The sternum or breast bone forms the anterior midline part of the bony thorax. Although embryologically it is made up of five elements, in the adult only three parts—the manubrium (upper part), body, and xiphoid process (lower part)—are recognized (Figure 3-2).

The manubrium is about 2 in. long and is usually described as shield shaped. It has an upper concavity called the jugular notch. Laterally and slightly inferior to the jugular notch are the clavicular notches for articulations with the clavicle. Laterally below the clavicular notch is a depression for articulation with the first costal cartilage. The manubrium articulates with the body, which is somewhat longer and shaped much like a beaver's tail. Along its lateral margin, the body of the sternum has numerous depressions for articulation with the second to seventh costal cartilage.

Inferiorly is the small, highly variable xiphoid process. It serves mainly as a point of attachment for the linea alba and for some of the muscles of the anterior abdominal wall. It may be palpated in the apex of the infrasternal angle.

The bony thorax has an upper aperture referred to as the thoracic inlet. The thoracic inlet is bounded by the body of the first thoracic vertebra, first rib and costal cartilage, and manubrium sterni. Many structures such as the esophagus, trachea, jugular vein, and great arteries enter and leave the thoracic cavity through the thoracic inlet.

The lower end of the thoracic cage is known as the thoracic outlet. It is wider in diameter than the thoracic inlet and is bounded by the body of the twelfth thoracic vertebra, lower six costal cartilages, and twelfth rib on either side. The outlet is usually closed by the diaphragm, which is a dome-shaped muscle that rises to the level of the fifth or sixth rib. A description of the diaphragm is given below.

Articulations

The head and tubercle of the ribs are attached to the thoracic vertebrae by synovial joints. The other end of the ribs articulates

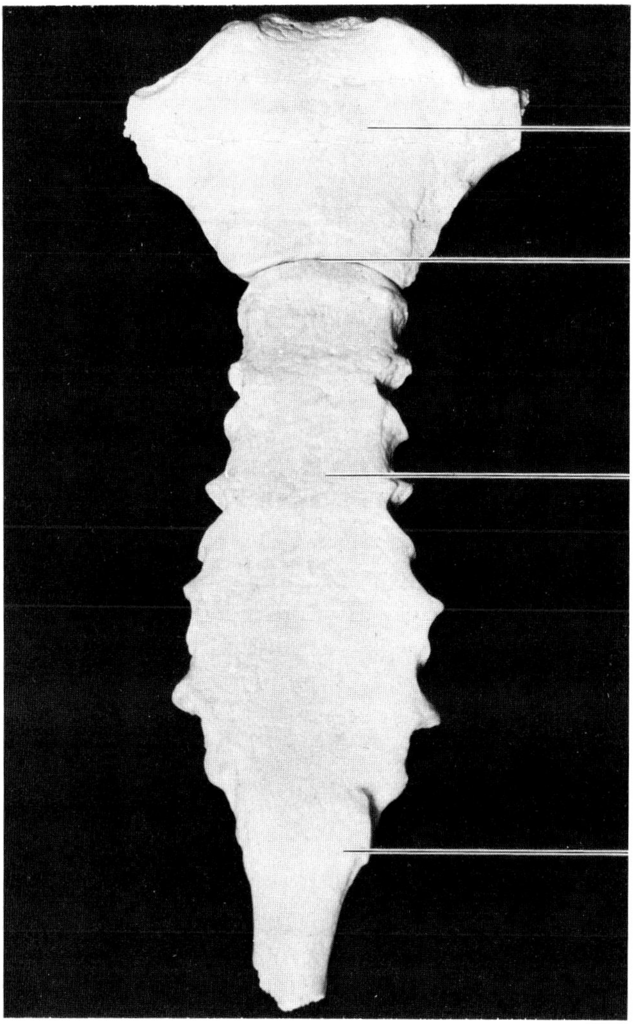

Figure 3-2. Sternum

with the sternum through the costal cartilage. This is a synchondrosis that permits a small amount of movement. Because of this arrangement, movement of the thoracic cage is possible during respiration. By the action of the associated muscles, the ribs are raised and lowered during inspiration and expiration.

THORACIC MUSCLES

Numerous muscles are attached to the thoracic cage, and they may be divided into two groups: the extrinsic and intrinsic muscles. The extrinsic muscles are muscles of the head, back, abdomen, and upper limb that are partly or totally attached to the thoracic cage. Although these muscles play an auxiliary role in respiration, especially forced respiration, their major function is the movement of the head, neck, and so on.

The intrinsic muscles are those attached wholly to the bones of the thorax and are intimately associated with respiration. Although the diaphragm (to be discussed later) is generally regarded as the major muscle of respiration, the intrinsic thoracic muscles assist in the raising and lowering of the ribs, resulting in increased and decreased thoracic volume. The intrinsic muscles will be described below.

Intrinsic Muscles of the Thorax

EXTERNAL INTERCOSTALS

There are 11 pairs of external intercostal muscles located in the 11 intercostal spaces. Each muscle extends from the lower border of the rib above to the upper border of the rib below. The fibers of the muscle rub obliquely downward and forward. Each muscle extends from the angle of the rib posterolaterally to the junction of the rib and its costal cartilage anteriorly. The remaining space between the costal cartilages up to the sternum is occupied by the external intercostal membrane.

INTERNAL INTERCOSTALS

There are also 11 pairs of internal intercostal muscles. These muscles are deep to the external intercostals, and although the attachments are the same, the fibers are oriented at right angles to the external intercostals (i.e., they run downward and backward). Each muscle extends from the sternum anteriorly to the angle of the rib. The posterior intercostal membrane fills the gap between the posterior part of the rib and its attachment to the vertebrae.

INNERMOST INTERCOSTALS

The innermost intercostal muscles are highly variable and are not easily demonstrated. They are usually regarded as an inner layer of the internal intercostal muscle. Midway along the intercostal space, the internal intercostal muscles split into two layers, allowing the passage of blood vessels and nerves within the strata. The innermost layer is usually regarded as the innermost intercostal muscles.

SUBCOSTALS

The subcostal muscles are seen on the internal surface of the thorax. Their number, size, and shape vary. Usually they are found on the internal surface of the posterior wall of the thoracic cage. Their fibers run in the same direction as the internal intercostal muscles, but they span more than one intercostal space.

TRANSVERSE THORACIC MUSCLES

The transverse muscles of the thorax are found on the internal surface of the anterior wall of the thoracic cage. Their slips of muscle fibers extend from the lower part of the sternum and are attached to the costochondral junction of the second to the sixth rib. The internal thoracic (mamillary) artery and vein run anterior to this muscle.

All of the above muscles are innervated by the associated intercostal nerve. Blood is supplied by way of the intercostal arteries, the internal thoracic arteries, and branches of the axillary artery on its anterolateral surface.

THE DIAPHRAGM

The diaphragm is usually regarded as the major muscle of respiration. It is an arched musculotendinous sheet that separates the thoracic from the abdominal cavity (Figure 3-3). Structures passing between the thorax and the abdomen pass through or behind the diaphragm. The circumferential part of the diaphragm is made up of muscle fibers that curve upward and inward to insert onto the ends of a connective tissue sheet called the central tendon. Several parts of the diaphragm are recognized.

Sternal Portion

The sternal portion is made up of two small slips of muscle fibers that arise from the posterior surface of the xiphoid process and insert onto the central tendon. On each side between it and the fibers of the costal portion is a small triangular gap, called the sternocostal triangle, that permits the passage of the superior epigastric vessels (the continuation of the internal thoracic vessels).

Costal Portion

The costal portion is the most extensive portion of the diaphragm. The muscle fibers originate from the inner surfaces of the lower six ribs on each side and insert on the central tendon.

Lumbar Portion

The fibers of the lumbar portion originate from the medial and lateral arcuate ligaments, which are thickened bands of fascia covering the psoas major and quadratus lumborum muscle, respectively. There is an area over the left lateral arcuate ligament that is known as the lumbocostal trigone. In this area, the diaphragm is thin and apparently weak. Herniation of the abdominal viscera into the thoracic cavity may occur at this region.

Crura

Occasionally, the crura are included as part of the lumbar portion of the diaphragm. These start out as tendinous bands firmly attached to the anterior longitudinal ligament of the lumbar vertebrae. The fibers forming the crura course upward to insert on

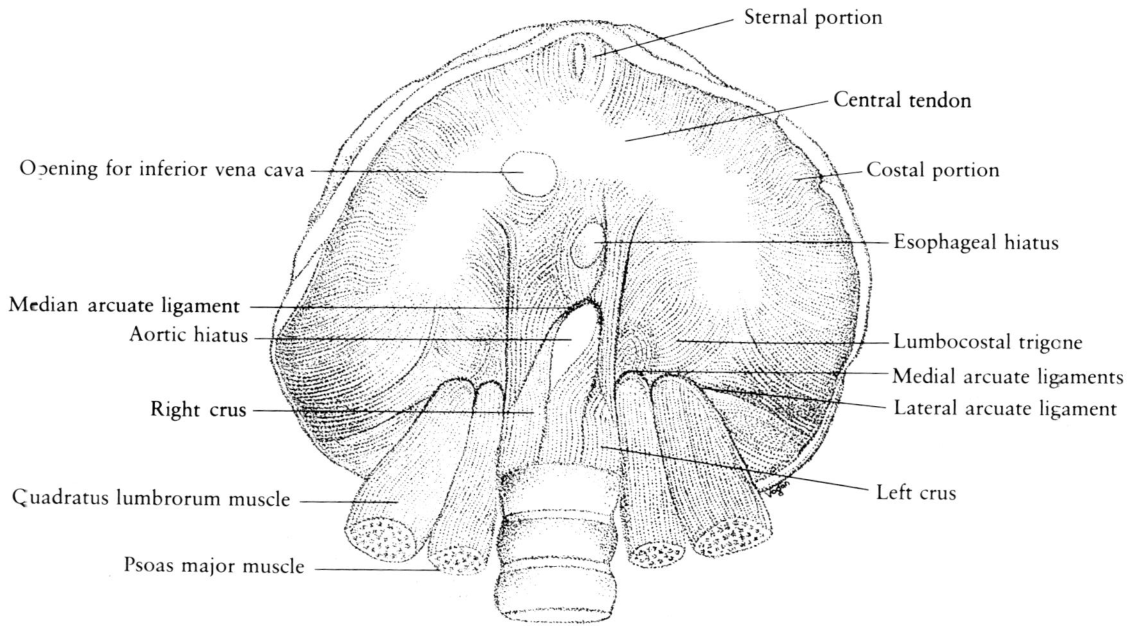

Figure 3-3. Diaphragm—viewed from below

trachea remains patent, and this is accomplished by the presence of between 16 to 20 C-shaped rings of hyaline cartilage that form the framework of the trachea. This arrangement ensures an open tube for the passage of air. The structure of the primary bronchi is similar to that of the trachea. After the bronchi enter the substance of the lungs and subdivide further, however, the cartilaginous rings are replaced by cartilaginous plates. There is a gradual reduction in the cartilaginous component as the bronchi further subdivide. By the time the subdivision reaches a diameter of 1 mm, no cartilage, only smooth muscle, is found in the wall of this tube, now called a bronchiole.

Bronchi

The right and left primary bronchi are the major divisions of the trachea. These two bronchi are not identical. The right bronchus is shorter, wider, and more vertical than the left (Figure 3-4). A foreign object entering the trachea is more likely to enter the right lung than the left. When the bronchi enter the lung, further subdivisions occur. Each primary bronchus divides into secondary bronchi (three on the right and two on the left), which supply the lobes of the lung. The secondary bronchi again subdivide such that there are 10 tertiary or segmental bronchi on each side. Each segmental bronchus supplies a bronchopulmonary segment.

The Lungs

The lungs are two light, spongy, elastic organs that, in the living state, are pink in color. Usually, the lungs in cadavers are seen to contain many dark granules which are the result of living in a polluted environment and inhaling dust particles and other pollutants. A smoker's lung is particularly contaminated by the carbon particles that are taken into the lungs when smoke is inhaled.

Each lung is covered by a double layer of mesothelial membrane known as the pleura. Between the layers of membrane is a potential space known as the pleural cavity. The lungs are attached to the bronchi and pulmonary vessels but are otherwise free within the thoracic cavity. They are not symmetrical. The right lung is divided into three lobes, whereas the left has only two. There is also a marked indentation on the lower medial aspect of the left lung that accommodates the heart. Each lung may be surgically divided into bronchopulmonary segments. A bronchopulmonary segment is usually defined as a segment of the lung that is supplied by a tertiary or segmental bronchus. This facilitates the removal of a segment or segments of the lung in diseased conditions, rather than removing a lobe or lobes as was previously done.

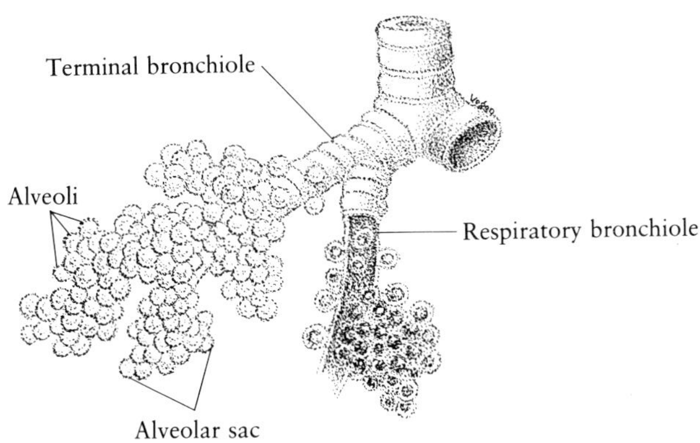

Figure 3-5. Respiratory tree

Within the bronchopulmonary segments, there is futher subdivision and specialization of the bronchioles leading to the alveolus. The respiratory unit of the lung begins with the terminal bronchiole. A schematic diagram of the final subdivisions of the respiratory tree is shown in Figure 3-5. Air in the alveolus is brought into close proximity to the blood in the rich capillary network that surrounds the alveolous, permitting gaseous exchange.

REVIEW QUESTIONS

1. Name the components of the bony thorax.
2. Name the parts of a typical rib.
3. Name the bones of the sternum.
4. List the intrinsic muscles of the thorax.
5. Describe the anatomy of the diaphragm.
6. Name the parts of the lower respiratory passage.
7. What are bronchopulmonary segments?
8. Where does gaseous exchange occur in the lung?

SUGGESTED READINGS

Crouch, J. E. *Functional Human Anatomy,* 3rd ed. Lea & Febiger, Philadelphia, 1978, pp. 135–140, 212–217.

Grant, J.C.B., and Basmajian, J.C. *Grant's Method of Anatomy,* 7th ed. Williams & Wilkins, Baltimore, 1965, pp. 463–474, 488–496.

Hollinshead, W.H. *Textbook of Anatomy,* 3rd ed. Harper & Row, New York, 1974, pp. 654–656.

4

Cavities of the Vocal Tract

The vocal tract is responsible for the generation and modification of speech sounds. The cavities of the vocal tract give speech its particular quality. Anatomically, there are four cavities. These are the buccal, oral, nasal, and pharyngeal cavities.

BUCCAL CAVITY

The buccal cavity is the smallest of the four cavities. It is highly variable in shape and dimensions and is limited by the lips and cheek externally and the teeth and gums internally. With the teeth clenched, the orifice between the lips communicates with the buccal cavity. The buccal cavity is also in communication with the oral cavity, with the jaws closed, by spaces between the teeth and the space on either side behind the last molars. It should also be noted that the duct bringing secretions from the parotid salivary gland opens into the buccal cavity. Its orifice is located on the inside of the cheek opposite the second upper molar.

ORAL CAVITY

The oral cavity is usually referred to as the cavity of the mouth. Anteriorly and laterally, it is bounded by the teeth and alveolar processes. Its superior limit is the hard and soft palate. The floor of the oral cavity is mainly muscular, the major constitutent being the tongue. Posteriorly, the oral cavity opens into the pharynx. The posterior boundary of the oral cavity is the anterior faucial pillars (palatoglossal arches). The posterior opening of the oral cavity is known as the fauces.

Fauces

The faucial opening may be regarded as the gateway between the oral cavity and pharynx. It has three boundaries. Superiorly, it is bounded by the soft palate. The palatoglossal and palatopharyngeal arches form the lateral margins of the fauces, and the dorsum of the tongue forms the inferior floor.

NASAL CAVITIES

The nasal cavities are two narrow symmetrical chambers separated by a nasal septum that bulges to one side, usually the right. It has contributions from several facial bones (see Chapter 1). The nasal cavities are in communication with the exterior of the body by way of the nostrils or anterior nares. Posteriorly, it is in communication with the pharynx through the posterior nares or conchae. The lateral wall of the nasal cavities is irregular and consists of three scroll-shaped bones called the superior, middle, and inferior conchae (Figure 1-2). The spaces between the bones are called meati (sing., meatus), and the parnasal sinuses and nasolacrimal duct empty into these spaces. In the roof of the nasal cavity is a specialized region of epithelium called the *olfac-*

tory epithelium, which subserves the sense of smell. Nerve fibers from the neurons in this epithelium pass through the cribriform plate of the ethmoid bone on their way to the olfactory bulbs on the base of the brain.

Inhaled air is warmed and filtered as it passes through the nasal cavity on its way to the lungs.

Paransal Air Sinuses

The paranasal air sinuses can best be visualized as air spaced within the frontal, ethomoid, sphenoid, and maxilla, and they bear the corresponding name, that is frontal sinuses, ethmoid sinuses, and so on. They are all in communication with the nasal cavity through the nasal meati. The mucuous membrane lining the nasal cavity is continuous with that lining the paranasal sinuses, nasopharynx, and pharyngotympanic tube. It is a thin membrane that is closely attached to the underlying periosteum and perichondrium. Structurally, it consists of pseudostratified, ciliated, columnar epithelium with numerous goblet cells, resting on a basement membrane. The underlying connective tissue is rich in blood vessels and lymphocytes and contains spaces next to the periosteum that become dilated as a result of irritation. This is responsible for the fullness felt in the head and face during infection, from colds, sinusitis, and the like.

The role of the paranasal sinuses is unclear. However, it is believed that they subserve two functions: (1) the air spaces in the bones cause a reduction in the weight of the bones of the face; and (2) they must play a role in voice resonance, since any changes in the sinuses have a marked effect on the quality of the voice.

THE PHARYNX

The pharynx is a musculofibrous tube that is suspended from the base of the skull and extends down to the level of the sixth cervical vertebra, where it is continuous with the esophagus. It serves as a common passageway for food and air and communicates with the nasal cavity, oral cavity, and larynx. The areas of the pharynx opposite these cavities are known as the nasopharynx, oropharynx, and laryngopharynx, respectively. The pharynx is open anteriorly but closed laterally and posteriorly. The posterior wall is separated from the cervical vertebrae by a thin layer of fascia and a potential space. The lateral walls are related to the styloid process and its muscles, as well as to the nerves and great vessels of the neck.

The Wall of the Pharynx

The pharyngeal wall consists of four coats.

THE MUCOSA

The mucosa is the innermost coat and consists of a lining that is a ciliated, pseudostratified, columnar epithelium in the nasopharynx but changes to stratified squamous in the region of the oropharynx and laryngopharynx. Below the epithelium in the submucosa are mucous glands, lymphoid tissue, and venous plexuses.

FIBROUS COAT

The fibrous coat is a relatively tough fibrous membrane that, because of its attachments, helps to maintain the patency of the pharynx. Superiorly, it is firmly attached to the base of the skull from the root of the median pterygoid plate to the median pharyngeal tubercle of the basioccipital bone. Anteriorly, it is attached to the medial pterygoid palate. The pharyngobasila fascia is best seen, in the region superior to the superior constrictor muscle, just below its attachment to the base of the skull.

MUSCLE COAT

There are six muscles associated with the pharynx. Three of these, the stylopharyngeus, palatopharyngeus, and salpingopharyngeus elevate the pharynx and larynx during deglutition. The other three are the constrictor muscles and are named for their location. They are the superior, middle, and inferior constrictors (Figure 4-1). The extent and action of these muscles are summarized in Table III.

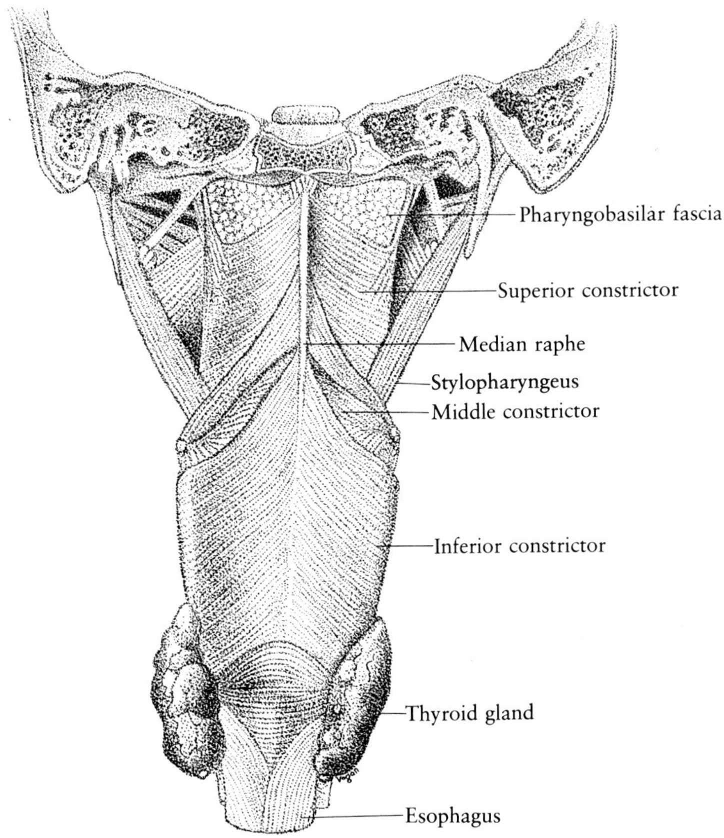

Figure 4-1. Pharyngeal muscles—from behind

Table III. Muscles of the pharynx

Name	*Origin*	*Insertion*	*Nerve Supply*	*Action*
Superior constrictor	1. Posterior border of medial pterygoid lamina 2. Pterygomandibular raphe 3. Mylohyoid ridge of mandible 4. Side of tongue	1. Pharyngeal tubercle at base of skull 2. Median raphe	Accessory	Constricts
Middle constrictor	Hyoid bone and stylohyoid ligament	Median raphe	Accessory	Constricts
Inferior constrictor	Outer surface of thyroid cartilage and cricoid cartilage	Median raphe	Accessory	Constricts
Stylopharyngeus	Root of styloid process	Posterior border of thyroid cartilage and wall of pharynx	Glossopharyngeal	Elevates pharynx and larynx
Palatopharyngeus	Upper surface of palatal aponeurosis	Side of pharynx and posterior border of thyroid cartilage	Accessory	Elevates, also constricts isthmus
Salpingo pharyngeus	Medial end of cartilaginous pharyngotympanic tube	Inserts with palatopharyngeus	Accessory	Similar to above

BUCCOPHARYNGEAL FASCIA

The outermost covering of the pharynx is a thin layer of loose areolar connective tissue that surrounds the tube. It extends anteriorly over the cheek to cover the buccinator muscle and is continuous below with the pretracheal fascia.

Cavities of the Pharynx

NASOPHARYNX

The nasopharynx is the uppermost part of the pharynx that is in communication anteriorly with the nasal cavity. Its roof is made up of the sphenoid bone, and its posterior wall is muscular. There is a mass of lymphoid tissue located in the roof and posterior walls known as the pharyngeal tonsils or adenoids. The lateral walls are also muscular and contain the openings of the pharyngotympanic tube. The superior and posterior lips of the opening of the pharyngotympanic tube are thickened because of the underlying cartilage and are surrounded by aggregations of lymphoid tissue known as the tubal tonsils. Passing inferiorly from the posterior lip of the tubal orifice is the salpingopharyngeal fold overlying the salpingopharyngeus muscle which will insert on the thyroid cartilage (see Table III). Superior to this fold is a depression known as the pharyngeal recess.

OROPHARYNX

The oral cavity opens into the oropharynx. Its upper limit is the soft palate, and its lower limit is opposite the posterior one third of the tongue. The faucial pillars are located on either side of the opening of the oral cavity. Two arches make up the faucial pillars. Anteriorly is the palatoglossal arch, which is made up of the palatoglossal muscle and its covering mucosa. Posteriorly is the palatopharyngeal arch. Between the two arches is a space known as the tonsillar fossa containing the palatine tonsils.

LARYNGOPHARYNX

The laryngopharynx lies posterior to the larynx and extends from the upper edge of the epiglottis down to the pharyngoesophageal junction. The inlet of the larynx lies in the median part of its anterior wall. On either side of the laryngeal opening lie the deep piriform recesses. The cavity of the laryngopharynx is relatively narrow, being shaped like a curved slit with an anterior concavity. Inferiorly, the laryngopharynx is continuous with the esophagus.

Blood Supply

The pharynx is supplied by branches from the external carotid artery, primarily the ascending pharyngeal artery and the facial artery. Venous drainage is to the pharyngeal plexus and thence to the internal jugular vein. Deep cervical nodes provide for lymphatic drainage of this area. Pharyngeal infections usually are accompanied by enlarged lymph nodes in the neck ("swollen glands").

Nerve Supply

The pharyngeal plexus of nerves along with the pharyngeal venous plexus is located on the posterior surface of the middle constrictor muscle. The nerve plexus receives branches from the vagus, accessory, and glossopharyngeal nerves, as well as from the superior cervical sympathetic ganglion. Sensory innervation of the pharynx is by way of the branches from the glossopharyngeal nerves. The accessory nerve provides motor innervation of the muscles of the pharynx, except for the stylopharyngeus, which is supplied by a motor branch of the glossopharyngeal. The muscles of the soft palate are also supplied by the accessory nerve, except for the tensor veli palatini, which is supplied by a branch of the mandibular division of the trigeminal nerve. The sympathetic fibers pass into the smooth muscle of the blood vessels of the pharynx and to its mucous glands.

DEGLUTITION

Deglutition, or the act of swallowing, is accomplished by the actions of the tongue, palate, pharynx, and larynx. These structures are acted upon by their respective muscles to form the bolus and pass it into the esophagus. There are two phases of deglutition, a voluntary stage followed by an involuntary one.

The Voluntary Stage

After mastication, the tongue forces the bolus up against the hard palate toward the posterior part of the oral cavity. The soft palate closes down on the back of the tongue and helps to form the bolus. At the same time, the hyoid bone is moved forward and upward, where it is fixed by the action of the geniohyoid, mylohyoid, digastric, and stylohyoid muscles. The posterior part of the tongue is drawn upward by the styloglossus muscles, and the palatoglossus muscles contract to approximate the palatoglossal arches. The bolus then passes through the oropharyngeal isthmus (fauces) into the oropharynx, where the involuntary phase is initiated.

The Involuntary Stage

With the bolus in the oropharynx, the soft palate is elevated and tightened by the actions of the levator veli palatini and tensor veli palatini muscles. Because of this action and the combined actions of the pharyngeal sphincter and superior pharyngeal constrictor muscle, the soft palate is closely approximated to the pharyngeal wall. This prevents the bolus from passing upward into the nasopharynx. At the same time, through the actions of the stylopharyngeus, salpingopharyngeus, palatopharyngeus, and thyrohyoid muscles, the larynx is drawn up behind the hyoid bone and the pharynx with it. The entrance to the larynx is essentially closed and protected as a result of the action of the aryepiglottic, oblique arytenoids and thyroarytenoid muscles. Partly by gravity and partly by the contractions of the superior and middle pharyngeal constrictors, the bolus slips over the larynx into the lower pharynx. The palatopharyngeus muscle contracts again, pulling the pharynx up, and at the same time the inferior pharyngeal constrictor contracts to push the bolus into the esophagus. It is then propelled down the esophagus by peristalsic waves of contractions into the stomach.

REVIEW QUESTIONS

1. What are the boundaries of the buccal cavity?
2. What are the boundaries of the oral cavity?
3. What is the fauces?
4. Name the paranasal air sinuses.
5. What structures are located on the lateral walls of the nasal cavities?
6. Name the four coats of the pharyngeal wall.
7. What are the gross divisions of the pharynx.
8. Name the six muscles of the pharynx and list their action.
9. Describe the processes that occur during deglutition.

SUGGESTED READINGS

Crouch, J.E. *Functional Human Anatomy,* 3rd ed. Lea & Febiger, Philadelphia, 1978, pp. 474–485.

Hollinshead, W.H. *Textbook of Anatomy,* 3rd ed. Harper & Row, New York, 1974, pp. 928–935.

5

Structures Associated with Articulation

FACIAL MUSCLES

The facial muscles are made up of two groups: (1) the muscles of facial expression and (2) the muscles of mastication. The muscles of facial expression will be considered first.

The pattern of distribution of the muscles of facial expression is shown in Figure 5-1. Generally, it can be said that there are muscles that surround the orifices, and these are connected to muscles that run vertically, horizontally, and angularly. The size, shape, and extent of the development of these muscles are variable and depend on age, sex, dentition, and individual variation. These muscles are also unique in that there are no discrete fascial sheaths as seen in other muscles. The muscles of facial expression insert directly into the skin. Functionally, all the muscles act as a unit, most of them acting on the lips, which are the most mobile

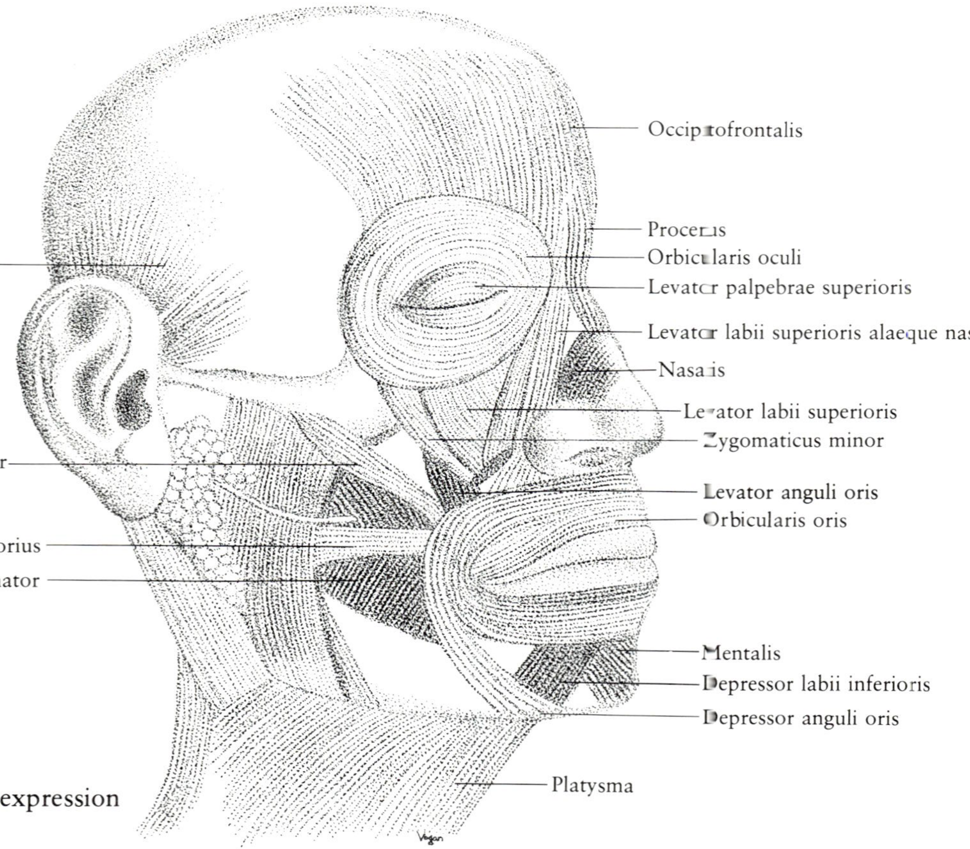

Figure 5-1. Muscles of facial expression

Table IV. Muscles of facial expression

Muscles of the scalp	Occipitofrontalis Temporoparietalis
Muscles of the eyelids	Levator palpebrae superioris Orbicularis oculi Corrugator supercilii
Muscles of the nose	Procerus Nasalis Depressor septi nasi
Muscles of the mouth	Levator labii superioris alaeque nasi Levator labii superioris Zygomaticus minor Zygomaticus major Levator anguli oris Mentalis Depressor labii inferioris Depressor anguli oris Buccinator Orbicularis oris Risorius

part of the face. Table IV lists the individual muscles. All the muscles of facial expression are innervated by the facial nerve.

The distribution of the branches of the facial nerve after it emerges from the stylomastoid foramen is shown in Figure 5-2. The five major branches of the facial nerve are the temporal, zygomatic, buccal (two parts), mandibular, and cervical branches. In addition, there is a small posterior auricular branch that leaves the nerve at the stylomastoid foramen and passes behind the auricle of the ear to supply some muscles of the auricle and the occipital part of the occipitofrontalis muscle.

Damage to the facial nerve may lead to paralysis of the muscles of the face. The most common type is Bell's palsy, which results from inflammation of the nerve close to the stylomastoid foramen. Its cause is uncertain. Depending on the extent of the damage to the nerve, there is generally a loss of tonus of the affected muscles and a drooping of the facial structures on the affected side. Closure of the eye is difficult, and the lips cannot be pursed. Dribbling of food occurs during eating. Speech is usually affected owing to the paralysis of the labial muscles. Most cases of Bell's

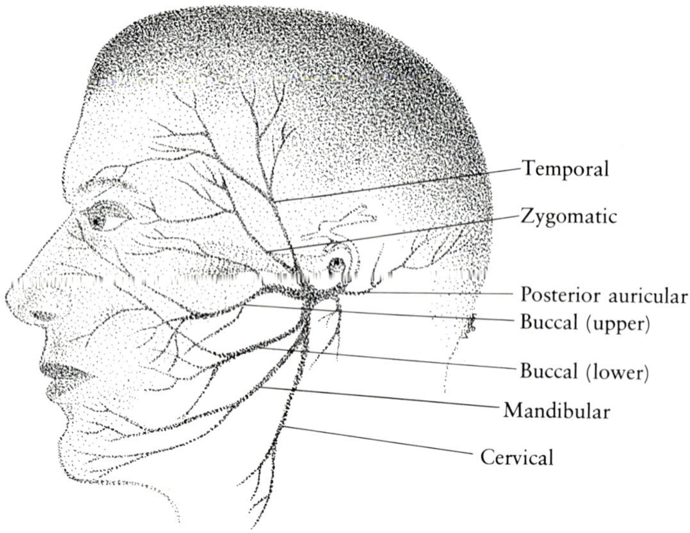

Figure 5-2. Branches of the facial nerve

palsy show some improvement after 10 days, and recovery is almost always complete.

MOUTH

The mouth is the most movable and adjustable part of the vocal tract. It comprises the teeth, hard palate, soft palate, and lower jaw associated with the lips, cheeks, and tongue. The lips and tongue are very mobile and play an important role in speech.

Lips

The lips constitute the orifice of the mouth. They are covered by skin externally and mucous membrane internally, with a layer of muscle and fat in between. The red area of the lips is called the vermillion area. It is covered by thin, nonkeratinized epithelium with a high content of eleidin. The blood vessels below the epithelium account for its reddish appearance. On the upper lip, there is a midline tubercle at the base of the philtrum. On the internal surface, there is a short band of tissue called the labial frenulum that attaches the lip to the alveolar process of the upper jaw (maxilla). There is a small frenulum on the lower lip, but it is not as prominent. Below the mucosa, on the inner surface of the lips, there are labial glands that serve to keep the lips moist. The muscles of the lips are shown in Figure 5-1.

Cheeks

The cheeks from the lateral wall of the mouth and buccal cavity. The structure is similar to the lips with skin externally, fat and muscles in the middle, and mucosa internally. Below the mucosa, there are buccal glands similar to the buccal glands described above. The skin in the cheeks is keratinized, unlike that found on the vermillion area of the lips. There is a prominent buccal fat pad (pad of Bichat) found below the skin. This pad is best seen in suckling infants. There are two groups of muscles in this area. These include some muscles of facial expression and two of the muscles of mastication. These muscles are described in Tables IV and VII.

The cavity of the mouth is usually moist during speech as a result of the secretions of the buccal glands and salivary glands. There are three pairs of salivary glands. The largest is the parotid gland, which is located anterior to and below the external auditory meatus (Figure 5-3). Its duct (Stensen's duct) crosses the masseter muscle to open on the inner surface of the cheek opposite the upper second molar. The other salivary glands are located in the floor of the mouth.

The submandibular gland lies partly under cover of the mandible and between the mandible and the hyoid bone. Its duct, the submandibular duct, emerges from the medial surface of the gland and passes deep to the adjacent sublingual gland to open on the sublingual papilla at the side of the frenulum linguae. The sublingual gland is the smallest salivary gland. It lies under the sublingual fold in the floor of mouth (Figure 5-3). From its upper surface, a series of about a dozen small ducts pierce the mucous membrane and pour their secretions into the floor of the mouth.

of the teeth in facial appearance, mastication, and speech, their proper care cannot be overemphasized.

Tongue

The tongue, located in the floor of the mouth, plays an important role in speech, mastication, and deglutition. Its role in speech is so important that damage or paralysis of the tongue severely interferes with the ability to pronounce words properly. The tongue may be described as an epithelial bag of muscles fixed at one end. The epithelium is of the stratified squamous type. Anatomically, the tongue is divided into two parts: (1) The *root* is the fixed part. Structures passing in and out of the tongue enter and leave through the root. Because of this arrangement, the root is connected to the mandible and hyoid bone. (2) The *body* is the highly mobile part of the tongue. This anatomical division is the result of the different embryological origins of the two parts of the tongue. The tongue is a very interesting organ from a developmental standpoint, and this aspect will be covered in detail in the section on embryology. The description of the tongue can be broken down into two parts—the dorsum and the inferior surface and sides.

DORSUM OF THE TONGUE

The dorsum is the upper surface of the tongue and extends from the tip to the epiglottis (Figure 5-5). It consists of two parts. The pharyngeal part is the upper portion of the root or posterior one third of the tongue, and the palatine part is located over the body or anterior two thirds. These parts are separated by a slight depression known as the sulcus terminalis.

Pharyngeal Part. The epithelial covering is smooth, thin, and nodular. The nodular appearance results from the presence of numerous lymphatic follicles in the underlying submucosa. This collection of follicles is known as the lingual tonsils.

Palatine Part. The epithelium covering the palatine part of the tongue is thick and rough as a result of the presence of numerous papillae. There is also a midline depression known as the longitudinal median sulcus (Figure 5-5).

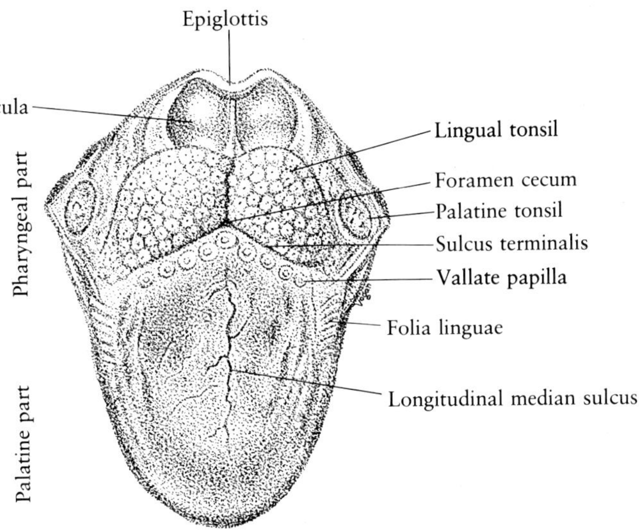

Figure 5-5. Dorsum of the tongue

Papillae. The papillae are microscopic projections on the tongue and may be divided into three types.

FILIFORM PAPILLAE The filiform papillae are the most numerous. They are minute, sharp-pointed projections that are distributed extensively over the dorsum of the tongue. They do not contain taste buds, and their major function appears to be to assist in gripping food. It should be noted that these papillae are highly developed in lower mammals that have very rough tongues, such as cats.

FUNGIFORM PAPILLAE Fungiform papillae are scattered over the dorsum and sides of the tongue. They are quite numerous on the tip and sides. These are mushroom-shaped structures that contain taste buds.

VALLATE OR CIRCUMVALLATE PAPILLAE The vallate or circumvallate papillae are the largest seen on the tongue. They range in number from 7 to 12 and are arranged in a row just anterior to the sulcus terminalis. They may best be visualized as being in the form of a small cylinder surrounded by a moat. Taste buds are located on the cylinder as well as in the wall of the moat.

INFERIOR SURFACE AND SIDES OF THE TONGUE

The mucous membrane covering the inferior surface and sides of the tongue is thin and smooth. Certain important structures may be seen on the underside of the tongue. Anteriorly in the midline is the frenulum linguae, which is a fold of mucous membrane that attaches the mobile part of the tongue to the floor of the mouth. Occasionally, this structure may be too short, leading to restricted mobility of the tongue and a speech impediment (tongue-tie) in children. Bilateral to the frenulum are the deep lingual veins. These are easily seen and are the venous return from the tip of the tongue. Two other structures—the sublingual papilla and the sublingual folds—may also be identified. The sublingual papilla is the site of opening of the duct of the submandibular salivary gland. The sublingual fold marks the course of this duct. The ductule of the sublingual gland opens along these folds.

On the sides of the tongue are three or four irregular folds known as the folia linguae (Figure 5-5). These, although well developed in lower animals, are vestigial in human beings.

MUSCLES OF THE TONGUE

The muscles of the tongue may be divided into two groups, intrinsic and extrinsic muscles. The intrinsic muscles are those that are contained within the epithelial bag, so to speak. They are named mainly on the basis of the orientation of their fibers. The extrinsic muscles, on the other hand, originate outside of the tongue, either on the hyoid bone or on the floor of the mouth (Figure 5-6). The fibers of these muscles enter the tongue through the root. The location and action of the muscles of the tongue are summarized in Table V. All the muscles of the tongue are innervated by the hypoglossal nerve, except for the palatoglossus muscle, which is innervated by the accessory nerve.

Other structures of the tongue that should be mentioned are the septum of the tongue and the glands. The septum is a median fibrous partition that runs from the tip of the tongue and is attached posteriorly to the hyoid bone. It does not reach the dorsum of the tongue, being separated from it by the superior longitudinal muscle. There are several small serous and mucous

Table V. Muscles of the tongue

Name	*Location*	*Action*
Intrinsic muscles		
Superior longitudinal	Under mucosa of tongue from tip to back	Curls tip upwards and rolls it posteriorly
Inferior longitudinal	Lies one on each side in lower part of tongue; posterior fibers attached to hyoid bone	Curls tip inferiorly and, acting with above, retracts and widens tongue
Transverse	Extends from median septum to margin of tongue	Narrows tongue and increases its height
Vertical	Extends from dorsum inferolaterally to sides	Flatten tongue; acting with transverse, increases its length
Extrinsic muscles		
Genioglossus	Fan shaped; extends from upper mental spine and radiates throughout length of tongue	Protrudes tongue; also depresses tongue during sucking
Styloglossus	Slender; extends from tip of styloid process and stylohyoid ligament to side of tongue in its whole length	Draws tongue upward and backward during swallowing
Hyoglossus	Arises from body and greater horn of hyoid bone and is inserted into the posterior half of side of tongue	Depresses tongue to produce a cavity in mouth during sucking
Palatoglossus	From inferior surface of palatal aponeurosis to posterolateral part of tongue	Depresses soft palate; elevates posterior part of tongue

Note. All the muscles of the tongue, except for the palatoglossus, are supplied by the hypoglossal nerve. The palatoglossus is supplied by the accessory nerve.

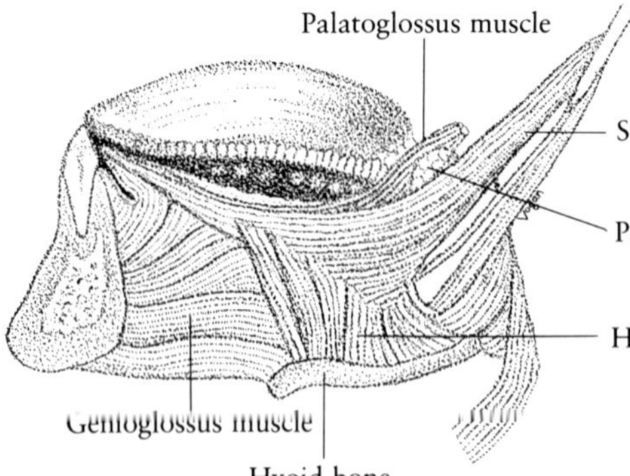

Figure 5-6. Tongue—extrinsic muscles

glands that lie below the mucosa of the pharyngeal part of the tongue, the tip, and the sides. There are also some serous glands that lie adjacent to the vallate papillae and open into the moat. On the inferior surface of the tongue near the tip are the so-called lingual glands. These are mixed mucous and serous glands that open by three or four ducts on the undersurface of the tip of the tongue.

BLOOD SUPPLY

The major blood supply to the tongue is derived from the lingual artery. This artery is a branch of the external carotid artery and arises near the greater horn of the hyoid bone. It enters the substance of the tongue near the anterior border of the hyoglossus muscle and follows a sinuous source to the tip of the tongue (Figure 5-7). Its major branches are as follows: 1. the dorsalis linguae branches supply the pharyngeal part of the tongue, pillars of the fauces, and the tonsils; 2. a sublingual branch supplies the sublingual gland, the mucosa of the floor of the mouth, and the gum on the inner surface of the lower jaw. The main branch that continues to the tip of the tongue is known as the profunda linguae artery. Venous return is by way of many venae comitantes. The major veins of the tongue are 1. the dorsal lingual veins, which accompany the dorsal lingual arteries and drain the

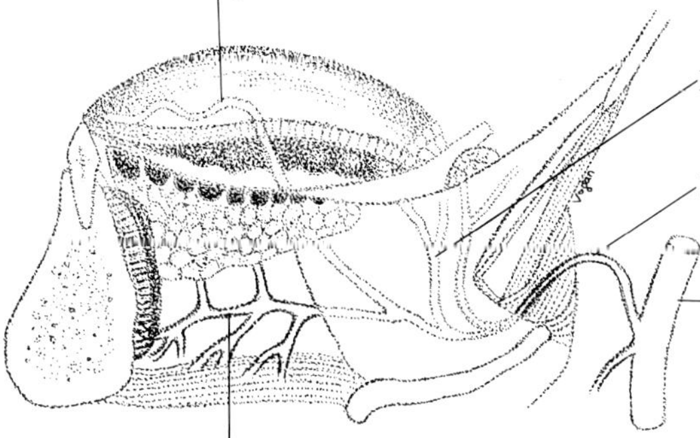

Figure 5-7. Tongue—blood supply

posterior one third of the tongue, and 2. the deep lingual veins, which drain the dorsum and sides of the tongue. These two vessals join with the deep sublingual vein to form the lingual vein, which enters the facial vein and which, in turn, empties into the internal jugular vein.

LYMPHATIC DRAINAGE

The tongue has a very extensive network of lymphatic vessels that empty into the equally extensive system of nodes seen in the floor of the mouth and neck. Generally, the pattern of drainage is as follows. The lymphatic vessels from the tip of the tongue drain into submental nodes and thence to the deep cervical nodes. There is also evidence of some drainage directly from the tip to the jugulo-omohyoid node. The body of the tongue is drained by the deep cervical nodes. The jugulodigastric nodes appear to be responsible for drainage of the root of the tongue. It should also be noted that there is no clear separation of the lymph plexuses on the right and left sides. Paramedian areas may drain equally to both sides.

NERVE SUPPLY

The tongue also has an extensive nerve supply which may be summarized as follows.

1. *Motor.* Hypoglossal nerve to all the muscles of the tongue except the palatoglossus, which is supplied by the accessory nerve.
2. *Sensory.*
   a. Lingual branch of the mandibular division of the trigeminal nerve: general sensation to the anterior two thirds of the tongue.
   b. Chorda tympani branch of the facial nerve, which runs in the sheath of the lingual nerve: taste sensation from the anterior two thirds of the tongue.
   c. Lingual branch of the glossopharyngeal nerve: taste and general sensation from the posterior one third of the tongue, including the vallate papillae.
   d. Twigs of the internal branch of the superior laryngeal nerve to a small area adjacent to the epiglottis: general sensation and taste from scattered taste buds in this region.

Most of the above nerves also carry parasympathetic secretomotor fibers to the glands in the tongue.

Palate

The palate forms the upper limit of the oral cavity. It consists of two parts, the hard palate anteriorly and the soft palate posteriorly. The hard palate is made up of bony contributions from the maxilla and palatine bones. It is covered with a mucosa that has a stratified squamous epithelium and submucosal mucous glands. The soft palate is attached to the posterior end of the hard palate and is made up of a connective tissue core (palatine aponeurosis) covered by muscles and an overlying mucosa. In the midline, there is a small projection of tissue that hangs down. This is called the uvula. The palate plays an important role in speech, and defects in the palate (e.g., clefts) cause speech abnormalities. The palate also plays an important role in deglutition, with the soft palate closing off the nasopharynx and preventing food from entering therein. The muscles of the soft palate are summarized in Table VI. Because of the attachments of the palatoglossus and palatopharyngeus muscles, they are also included in considering the muscles of the tongue and palate as well.

Table VI. Muscles of the soft palate

Muscle	*Origin*	*Insertion*	*Action*	*Nerve Supply*
Palatoglossus	Inferior surface of palatine aponeurosis	Sides of tongue	Raises the tongue and narrows the fauces	Pharyngeal branch of the accessory nerve
Palatopharyngeus	Posterior border of hard palate and upper surface of palatine aponeurosis	Posterior border of thyroid cartilage	Elevates the larynx and tenses the soft palate	Pharyngeal branch of the accessory nerve
Musculus uvulae	Posterior nasal spine	Mucosa of uvula	Closes the nasopharynx	Pharyngeal branch of the accessory nerve
Levator veli palatini	Inferior surface of petrous bone and medial part of auditory tube	Palatine aponeurosis	Elevates the soft palate	Pharyngeal branch of the accessory nerve
Tensor veli palatini	Posterior end of medial pterygoid plate and lateral surface of auditory tube	Palatine aponeurosis and posterior border of hard palate	Tenses the soft palate, opens eustachian tube	Mandibular nerve

TEMPOROMANDIBULAR JOINT

Although movement at the temporomandibular joint is not very obvious during phonation, the integrity of this joint is important in voice production. Restricted movement at this joint resulting from any type of abnormality usually has a marked effect on speech production. It should also be recalled that the maxilla bears the upper teeth and the mandible the lower. Many important sounds are produced by the interplay of the tip of the tongue with the backs of the teeth as well as by the space between the teeth. Major movements occur at the temporomandibular joint during chewing or yawning, and the muscles (of mastication) responsible for these actions are the same muscles that are active during speech.

The temporomandibular joint is a synovial joint in which the head of the condyloid process of the mandible articulates with the mandibular fossa of the temporal bone (Figure 5-8). These

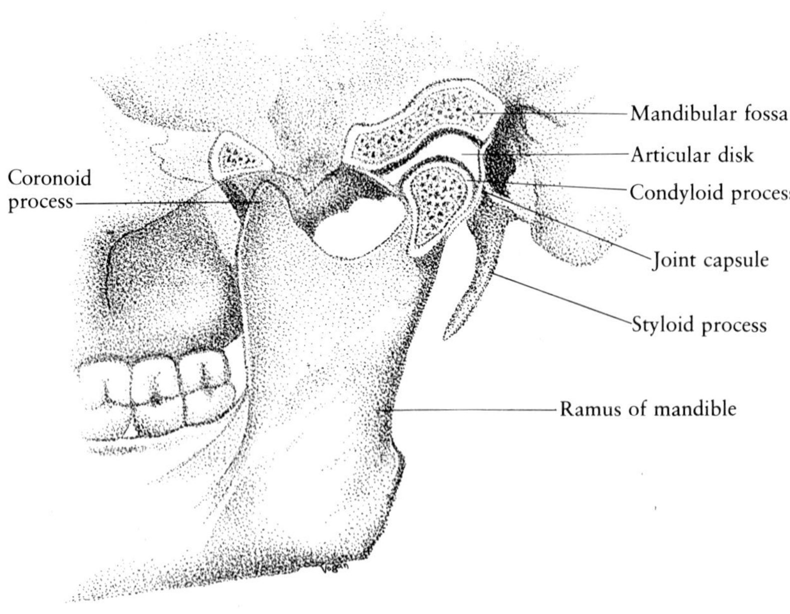

Figure 5-8. Temporomandibular joint—lateral view

bones are held together by a lax capsule that is strengthened by lateral thickenings of the capsule known as the temporomandibular ligament. Within the capsule, there is an articular disk that caps the head of the condyloid process. The disk divides the cavity into upper and lower joint compartments. This arrangement permits two types of movement. When the mandible is slightly depressed, a hinge movement is effected, and only the lower joint compartment is used. However, when the mouth is opened wide, as in yawning, the upper compartment, which permits the head of the condyloid process to glide anteriorly toward the articular spine, is also active (Figure 5-8). These movements may be investigated by palpating the joint located just anterior to the external auditory meatus and opening and closing the mouth.

This joint is relatively weak, the integrity of which is maintained mainly by the muscles of the mastication acting on the joint. In addition, however, there are two ligaments that also help to support the joints. These are the stylomandibular and sphenomandibular ligaments. The stylomandibular ligament runs from the styloid process to the back of the ramus of the mandible. The sphenomandibular ligament extends from the spine of the sphenoid bone to the lingula on the inner surface of the mandible (Figure 5-9).

The muscles of mastication and their actions are summarized in Table VII. It should be emphasized that the masseter and temporalis muscles are the major muscles involved in chewing. However, fine movements of the lower jaw, such as those required during speech, are accomplished by the medial pterygoid muscle assisted to some extent by the lateral pterygoid muscle. The student is advised to use Table VII in combination with Figures 5-10, 5-11, and 5-12 to obtain an understanding of the relationship of these muscles.

HYOID BONE

The hyoid, a U-shaped bone, is located in the floor of the mouth and is completely embedded in muscle. It consists of a central body and two processes known as the greater cornu (horns). At the junction of the body and greater cornu on each side, there is a

Table VII. Muscles of mastication

Muscle	*Origin*	*Insertion*	*Action*
Masseter	Lower border and deep surface of zygomatic arch	Lateral surface of ramus and coronoid process of mandible	Raises mandible: superficial fibers also protrude and deep fibers retract mandible; major role in chewing
Temporalis	Floor of temporal fossa; temporal fascia	Borders and medial surface of coronoid process: anterior border of ramus of mandible	Raises mandible: posterior fibers retract mandible after protrusion; major role in chewing
Lateral pterygoid (two parts)	*Upper head:* infratemporal crest and infratemporal surface of greater wing of sphenoid *Lower head:* lateral surface of lateral pterygoid plate	Front of neck of mandible and of capsule of mandibular joint	Protrudes mandible and pulls it toward opposite side; the right and left muscles act alternately in chewing
Medial pterygoid (two parts)	*Superficial head* (small): mainly from maxillary tuberosity *Deep head* (large): medial surface of lateral pterygoid plate	Medial surface of angle and ramus of mandible behind the mylohyoid groove	Elevates mandible; protrudes and pulls it to opposite side—aids the lateral pterygoid muscle in chewing; minor role in chewing, major role in speech

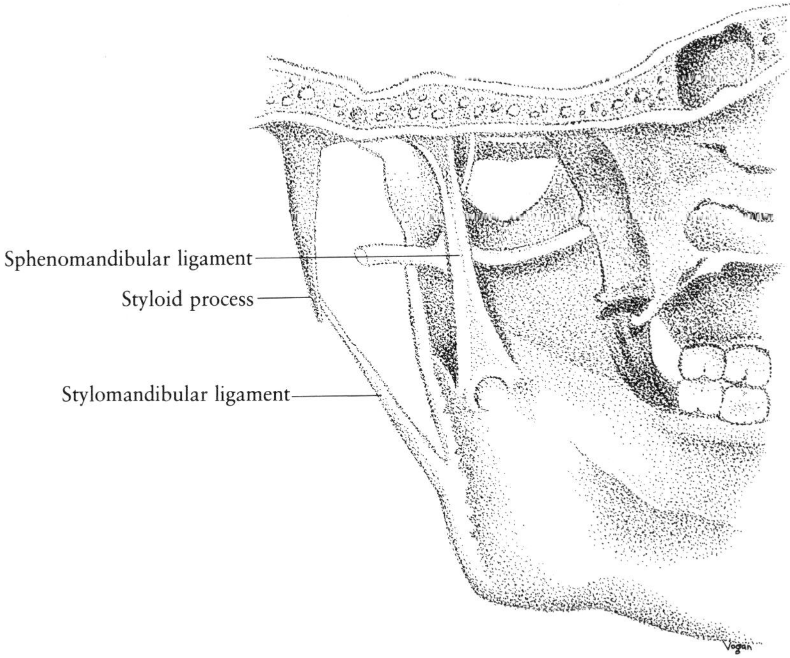

Figure 5-9. Temporomandibular joint—medial view

small upward projection known as the lesser cornu. The hyoid bone may be easily palpated in the neck just above the laryngeal prominence. It serves as the site of muscle attachment for many of the muscles of the floor of the mouth and front of the neck.

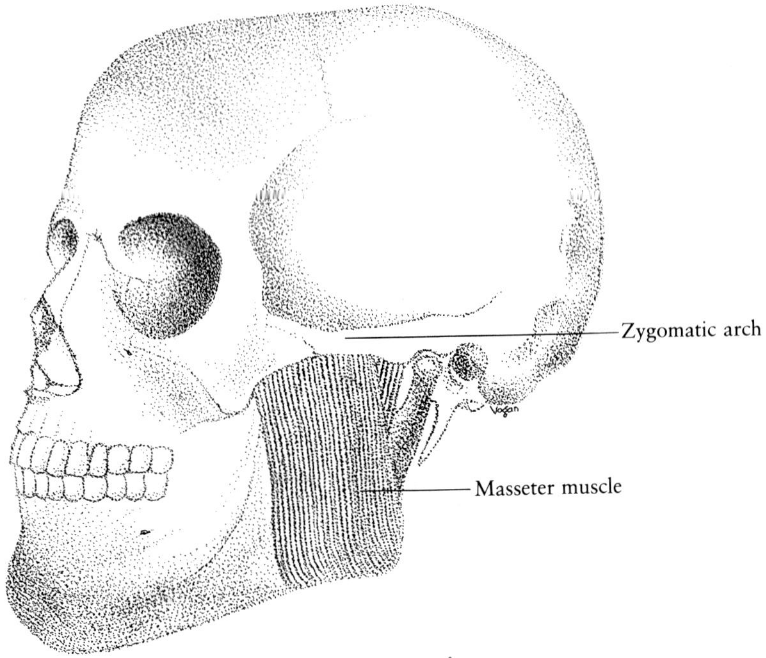

Figure 5-10. Masseter muscle

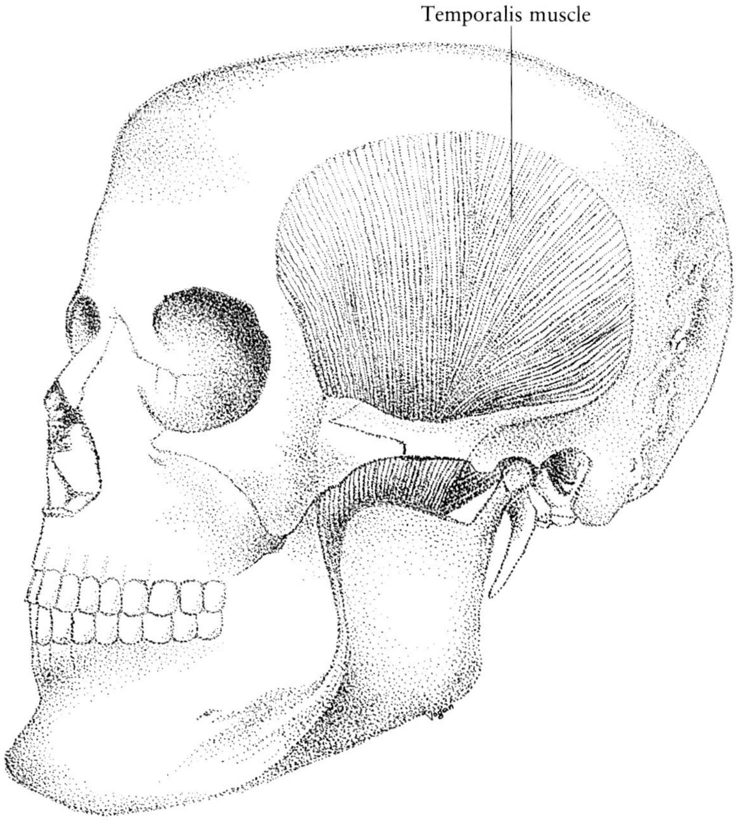

Figure 5-11. Temporalis muscle

6
The Larynx

CARTILAGES OF THE LARYNX

Thyroid Cartilage
Cricoid Cartilage
Epiglottis
Arytenoid Cartilages
Corniculate Cartilages
Cuneiform Cartilages

ARTICULATION OF THE LARYNX

Cricothyroid Joint
Cricoarytenoid Joint

MEMBRANES OF THE LARYNX

Extrinsic Laryngeal Membranes
THYROHYOID MEMBRANE
CRICOTHYROID MEMBRANE
Intrinsic Laryngeal Membranes
QUADRANGULAR MEMBRANE
CRICOVOCAL MEMBRANE

MUSCLES OF THE LARYNX

BLOOD SUPPLY AND INNERVATION OF THE LARYNX

CAVITY OF THE LARYNX

Upper Part

LARYNGEAL INLET

VESTIBULE

Middle Part

VESTIBULAR FOLDS

LARYNGEAL SINUS

VOCAL FOLDS

Lower Part

The larynx, or voice box, may be described as a musculocartilaginous hollow box located anteriorly in the neck. It is in close approximation to the hyoid bone above, being attached to it by suprahyoid muscles, and is continuous with the trachea below. It extends vertically across the third to the sixth cervical vertebrae, but its position may vary with age, sex, head position, and laryngeal activity. Some of its major functions are as follows: (1) it serves as a valve to regulate air entering and leaving the lungs, (2) it tends to prevent the entrance of foreign substances into the lungs and is capable of forcefully expelling such substances, and (3) it is capable of sound production.

The structures of the larynx may be broken down into three parts:

1. A cartilaginous framework consisting of the various laryngeal cartilages. This rigid framework serves to maintain an open airway, protects the superior aperture of the larynx, and is acted upon by muscles during vocalization.
2. Connective tissue that fills in the openings between the cartilages and are called membranes.
3. Muscles that act on the cartilages.

CARTILAGES OF THE LARYNX

The wall of the larynx is formed by three single cartilages (thyroid, cricoid, and epiglottis) and three paired small cartilages (arytenoid, corniculate, and cuneiform) held together by various membranes. The cartilages will be individually described.

Thyroid Cartilage

The thyroid cartilage is the largest cartilage and forms most of the anterior and lateral walls of the larynx. It is formed from two roughly quadrilateral plates of hyaline cartilage, called the lamina, which are fused anteriorly but separated posteriorly (Figure 6-1). The point of junction of the two laminae is known as the

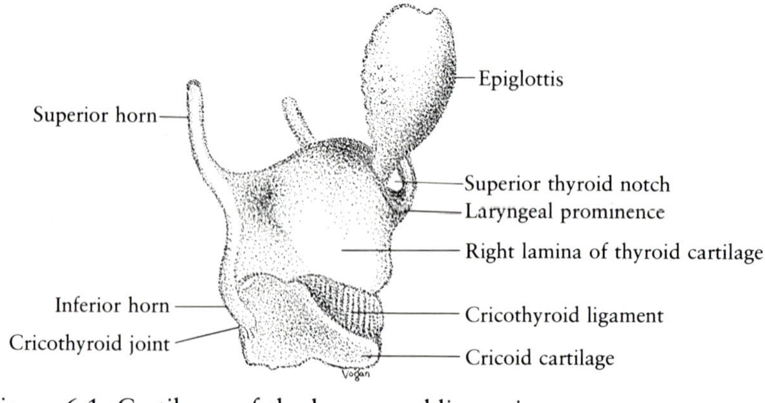

Figure 6-1. Cartilages of the larynx—oblique view

angle of the thyroid cartilage. There is a distinct notch at the superior end of this junction that is known as the superior thyroid notch. Just below this notch is the prominent anterior projection of the thyroid cartilage known as the laryngeal eminence or Adam's apple. This landmark is very prominent in males and may be easily palpated in the neck. Posteriorly, each lamina has an upward and downward projection known as the superior and inferior cornu (horn), respectively. The superior cornu is attached to the greater cornu of the hyoid bone, and the inferior cornu articulates with the cricoid cartilage. There are two major elevations on the lateral aspect of each thyroid lamina known as the superior and inferior tubercles. A slight elevation, joining these structures, is known as the oblique line, which serves as an important site for muscle attachment.

Cricoid Cartilage

The cricoid cartilage is thought to be shaped like a signet ring. It has an arch that is anterior and a lamina (the signet of the ring) posteriorly (Figure 6-2). It is located below the thyroid cartilage and articulates with the inferior cornus of the thyroid cartilage. Inferiorly, it is attached to the first tracheal ring by the cricotracheal membrane. There are several important landmarks on the cricoid cartilage. Laterally and somwhat inferiorly on the lamina on each side are depressions—articular facets for the inferior cornus of the thyroid cartilage. When viewed from the back, the lamina is seen to have a median ridge that separates two shallow depressions. The longitudinal muscles of the upper esophagus are attached to this ridge, and the posterior cricoarytenoid muscles occupy the depressions. At the top of the lamina is a midline depression, the posterior cricoid notch, which is flanked by two smooth convex articular facets that receive the bases of the arytenoid cartilages.

Epiglottis

This is a thin, leaflike structure made up of elastic cartilage (Figure 6-2). The narrow stem is attached on the inner side of the

MEMBRANES OF THE LARYNX

The membranes of the larynx may be divided into two groups: (1) the extrinsic laryngeal membranes, which connect the laryngeal cartilages to adjacent structures, and (2) the intrinsic membranes, which connect the cartilages with each other.

Extrinsic Laryngeal Membranes

THYROHYOID MEMBRANE

The thyrohyoid membrane is a fibroelastic sheet of connective tissue that connects the thyroid cartilage to the hyoid bone. It extends from the upper surface of the thyroid cartilage and is attached to the lower part of the body and greater horns of the hyoid bone (Figure 6-3). It is thickened in three areas. The anterior thickening is called the median thyrohyoid ligament. Laterally, the edge of the membrane, which extends between the superior horn of the thryroid cartilage and the tip of the major cornu

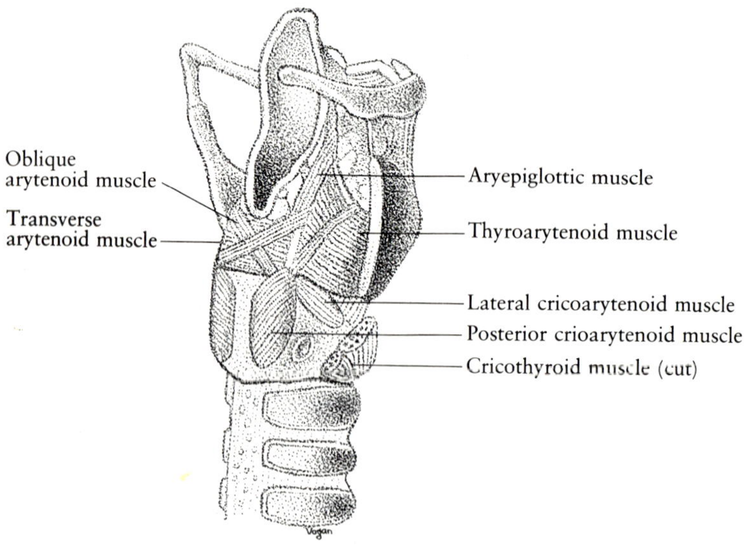

Figure 6-3. Intrinsic muscles of the larynx

of the hyoid bone, is round and almost cordlike and is known as the lateral thyrohyoid ligament. A cartilaginous nodule known as the cartilago triticea is located within this ligament.

The hyoepiglottic and thyroepiglottic ligaments were discussed earlier in connection with the epiglottis.

CRICOTRACHEAL MEMBRANE

The cricotracheal membrane attaches the lower border of the cricoid cartilage to the upper border of the first tracheal ring. It is slightly wider than the membrane that connects the subsequent tracheal rings with each other and is one of the sites used when a tracheotomy is performed.

Intrinsic Laryngeal Membranes

The intrinsic laryngeal membranes are generally thought to be one continuous sheet that lines the entire internal surface of the larynx and is called the elastic membrane of the larynx. It is covered for the most part by pseudostratified, ciliated, columnar epithelium, except over the vocal and vestibular ligaments. The mucosa overlying these structures has a stratified squamous epithelium. In the interest of simplicity of understanding and description, two distinct membranes will be described. These are the quadrangular and cricovocal membranes.

QUADRANGULAR MEMBRANE

The name of this paired membrane suggests its shape. The upper margin of each membrane is attached to the lateral margins of the epiglottis anteriorly and to the medial surface of the arytenoid cartilage posteriorly. This upper margin, along with its underlying muscle fibers of the aryepiglottic muscle is known as the aryepiglottic fold. The fibers of the quadrangular membrane course vertically. Its lower margin is attached anteriorly to the inside of the thyroid cartilage just below the thyroid notch. The posterior end of the lower margin is attached to the triangular fovea of the arytenoid cartilage. This lower margin is called the vestibular ligament. The vestibular ligament covered by mucosa is known as the vestibular fold or false vocal fold (Figure 6-4). The aryepiglottic

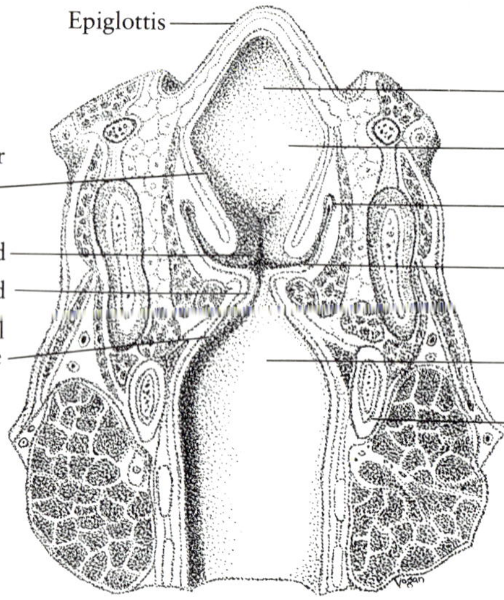

Figure 6-4. Coronal section of the larynx

folds surround the entrance to the larynx. The muscle that runs in the aryepiglottic fold (aryepiglottic muscle) is generally considered to be a continuation of fibers of the oblique arytenoid muscle. When the aryepiglottic muscles contract (e.g., during swallowing), they tend to close the gap between the aryepiglottic folds and at the same time pull the epiglottis over the opening. This prevents the passage of food and other substances into the larynx.

CRICOVOCAL MEMBRANE (CONUS ELASTICUS)

The cricovocal membrane originates on the superior border of the cricoid cartilage. Its fibers course medially and superiorly to a superior margin known as the vocal ligament (Figure 6-4). Anteriorly, the vocal ligament is attached to the thyroid cartilage just below the attachment of the vestibular ligament. Posteriorly, the vocal ligament is attached to the vocal process of the arytenoid cartilage. When covered by mucosa the vocal ligaments are referred to as the vocal folds or vocal cords. The cricovocal membrane is an elastic membrane that is thin laterally but thickened anteriorly to form the cricothyroid ligament, which extends from the superior border of the cricoid cartilage to the lower border of the thyroid cartilage. The thin lateral part of the cricovocal membrane is also referred to as the cricothyroid membrane.

MUSCLES OF THE LARYNX

The muscles acting on the laryngeal cartilages consist of two groups, the extrinsic and intrinsic muscle groups. The extrinsic muscles are those that act on the larynx as a whole, especially during swallowing. These muscles are located anteriorly in the neck and for simplicity are broken down into a suprahyoid and an infrahyoid group. Their extent and actions are summarized in Table VIII. It should be noted that the sternocleidomastoid, although located in the anterior neck, is not directly involved with the larynx. The intrinsic group of muscles are the muscles that act directly on the individual cartilages of the larynx and play a major role in speech Figure 6-3. The origin, insertion, and action of these muscles are also summarized in Table VIII.

BLOOD SUPPLY AND INNERVATION OF THE LARYNX

Blood is supplied to the larynx by way of the superior laryngeal branch of the superior thyroid artery and the inferior laryngeal branch of the inferior thyroid artery. The superior thyroid artery is a branch from the external carotid, whereas the inferior thyroid is from the thyrocervical trunk of the subclavian artery.

Motor innervation of the muscles of the larynx is effected by several nerves, namely the mandibular division of the trigeminal nerve, branches of the facial nerve, the accessory nerve, and the ansa cervicalis. These are summarized in Table VIII. The ansa cervicalis is a nerve loop located in the upper neck region formed from two roots. The upper root is a branch of the first cervical nerve, whereas the lower root is derived from the second and third cervical nerves. From this loop arise the branches that innervate the various muscles. Sensory innervation of the larynx comes from two sources. The internal laryngeal nerve supplies the mucosa down to the vocal folds, and the recurrent laryngeal nerve supplies the mucosa below this level.

Table VIII. Muscles of the neck

Muscle	*Attachments*	*Action*	*Innervation*
Suprahyoid group			
Digastric: Anterior belly	Chin area of mandible to hyoid bone	Together they depress mandible; if mandible is fixed, they elevate hyoid bone	Anterior: mandibular division of fifth cranial nerve
Posterior belly	Mastoid process to hyoid bone		Posterior facial nerve
Mylohyoid	Mylohyoid line of mandible and median raphe to hyoid bone	Elevates hyoid bone; tenses floor of mouth	Mandibular division of CV
Geniohyoid	Chin of mandible to hyoid bone	Elevates hyoid bone or depresses mandible	Ansa cervicalls
Stylohyoid	Styloid process to hyoid bone	Pulls up and back on hyoid bone	Facial nerve
Infrahyoid group			
Sternohyoid	Sternum to hyoid bone	Depresses hyoid bone	Ansa cervicalls
Sternothyroid	Sternum to oblique line of thyroid cartilage	Depresses thyroid cartilage	Ansa cervicalls
Thyrohyoid	Oblique line of thyroid cartilage to hyoid bone	Depresses hyoid bone or elevates thyroid cartilage	Ansa cervicalis
Omohyoid: Superior belly	Hyoid bone to intermediate tendon	Assists in depressing hyoid bone	Ansa cervicalls
Inferior belly	Intermediate tendon to scapula		
Associated muscle			
Sternocleido-mastoid	From clavicle and sternum to mastoid process	Pulls down on head	Accessory nerve

Table IX. Intrinsic laryngeal muscles

Muscle	*Origin*	*Insertion*	*Action*
Cricothyroid	Front and lateral surface of cricoid cartilage	Inferior horn and lamina of thyroid cartilage	Tenses vocal ligament
Posterior cricoarytenoid	Lower and medial part of lamina of cricoid cartilage	Back of muscular process of arytenoid cartilages	Abductor of vocal ligament
Lateral cricoarytenoid	Upper border of arch of cricoid cartilage	Front of muscular process of arytenoid cartilage	Adductor of vocal ligament
Transverse arytenoid	Back of muscular process and lateral border of one arytenoid cartilage	Corresponding parts on opposite arytenoid cartilage	Draws arytenoids together—closes rima glottidis
Oblique arytenoid	Back of muscular process of one arytenoid cartilage	Apex of other arytenoid cartilage	Draws arytenoids together—closes rima glottidis
Aryepiglottic	Some fibers of oblique arytenoid muscles continue around lateral sides over aryepiglottic folds on both sides		Shortens ary-epiglottic folds —closes inlet
Thyroarytenoid	Lower half of angle of thyroid cartilage and cricothyroid ligament	Anterolateral surface of arytenoid cartilage	Relaxes vocal folds
Vocalis	Deep slip of thyroarytenoid attached to lateral surface of vocal process and inferior impression on anterior surface of arytenoid cartilage; does not extend anteriorly to thyroid cartilage		Tightens segment of vocal ligament—high note
Thyroepiglottic	Some fibers of thyroarytenoid that run in aryepiglottic folds		Pulls epiglottis over larynx

Note. All of the above muscles are innervated by the recurrent laryngeal nerve on each side, except for the cricothyroid, which is innervated by a branch of the superior laryngeal nerve.

CAVITY OF THE LARYNX

A knowledge of the various chambers through which air passes on its way to and from the lungs and especially the structures it encounters in the larynx is useful for the understanding of sound production. The cavity of the larynx begins at the laryngeal inlet, which is in communication with the laryngopharynx and extends to the lower edge of the cricoid cartilage. This cavity may be divided into three parts Figure 6-4: 1. the upper part includes the laryngeal inlet and vestibule, 2. the middle part is bounded by vestibular and vocal folds, and 3. the lower part is located below the vocal folds.

Upper Part

LARYNGEAL INLET (ADITUS LARYNGIS)

The laryngeal inlet is the slitlike opening of the larynx and is located in a plane that is directed backward and upward. The opening is bounded anteriorly by the epiglottis, laterally by the aryepiglottic folds, and posteriorly by the interarytenoid fold. Contraction of the aryepiglottic muscles closes the aperture and pulls the epiglottis protectively over it.

VESTIBULE

The vestibule is the open cavity below the inlet. Its boundaries are similar to those of the inlet, and the vestibule extends down to the level of the vestibular folds.

Middle Part

VESTIBULAR FOLDS

The vestibular folds are thick pink folds of mucosa membrane that enclose a narrow band of fibrous tissue known as the vestibular ligament. The interval between the vestibular folds is known as the rima vestibuli. The vestibular folds are also called the false vocal cords.

LARYNGEAL SINUS (VENTRICLE)

The laryngeal sinus is a depression on the side wall between the vestibular and vocal folds. It extends almost the entire length of the vestibular folds. Extending from this cavity is a diverticulum of mucous membrane that is directed upward between the quadrangular membrane and the lamina of the thyroid cartilage. This structure is known as the saccule of the larynx. It contains numerous mucous glands that serve to keep the vocal folds moist.

VOCAL FOLDS

During examination of the larynx, the vocal folds appear as two white ridges just below and medial to the vestibular folds. Actually, they are the prominent free margins of the cricovocal membrane, with the overlying mucosa tightly bound down. The space between the vocal folds is called the rima glottidis (glottis) and is narrower than the rima vestibuli. The rima glottidis consists of two regions: 1. the intermembraneous region is the area between the vocal folds and makes up approximately three fifths of the length of the rima glottidis; 2. the second area is the intracartilaginous region, located between the arytenoid cartilages, and it accounts for the other two fifths of the length of the rima glottidis. During phonation, the space between the vocal folds is changed by the action of the intrinsic laryngeal muscles (see above).

Lower Part

Usually referred to as the infraglottal region, the lower part of the laryngeal cavity extends from the vocal folds to the lower border of the cricoid cartilage. There are no conspicuous features in this region, which is also known as the infraglottic cavity.

REVIEW QUESTIONS

1. List the cartilages of the larynx.
2. What is the laryngeal prominence (Adam's apple)?
3. What is the quadrangular membrane? To what structures is it attached?

4. Describe the cricovocal membrane.
5. List the suprahyoid group of extrinsic laryngeal muscles.
6. List the infrahyoid group of extrinsic laryngeal muscles.
7. List the intrinsic laryngeal muscles and give their innervation and action.
8. What are the vestibular folds?
9. What is the laryngeal sinus?
10. What are the vocal folds?

SUGGESTED READINGS

Crouch, J. E. *Functional Human Anatomy,* 3rd ed. Lea & Febiger, Philadelphia, 1978, pp. 521–524.

Hollinshead, W. H. *Textbook of Anatomy,* 3rd ed. Harper & Row, New York, 1974, pp. 939–948.

Zemlin, W. R. *Speech and Hearing Science.* Prentice-Hall, Englewood Cliffs, N.J., 1968, pp. 113–157.

7
Embryology

PHARYNGEAL APPARATUS

Pharyngeal Arches
Pharyngeal Clefts
Pharyngeal Pouches

FLOOR OF THE PHARYNX

Tongue
BODY OF THE TONGUE
ROOT OF THE TONGUE
MUSCLES OF THE TONGUE
Epiglottis
Thyroid Gland
Salivary Glands
SUBMANDIBULAR GLAND
SUBLINGUAL GLAND
PAROTID GLAND

DEVELOPMENT OF THE FACE

Nose and Primary Palate
Upper Part of the Face
Formation of the Palate

DEVELOPMENT OF THE EAR

External Ear
Middle Ear
Internal Ear

PHARYNGEAL APPARATUS

The pharyngeal apparatus consists of a series of mounds of tissue known as arches that are separated by depressions called clefts and pouches. These pharyngeal arches appear early in the fourth week of development as rounded elevations on the lateral sides of the cranial end of the embryo and surrounds the cranial part of the foregut (primitive pharynx). At this stage, four pairs of arches are clearly recognizable, and a fifth pair may be seen occasionally (Figure 7-1). The arches are separated from each other by depressions in the surface ectoderm known as pharyngeal clefts. Each arch and cleft is labeled in a craniocaudal sequence (Figure 7-1). Within the primitive pharynx, there is a series of depressions on the lateral walls that correspond to the invaginations of the pharyngeal clefts. These depressions, known as pharyngeal pouches,

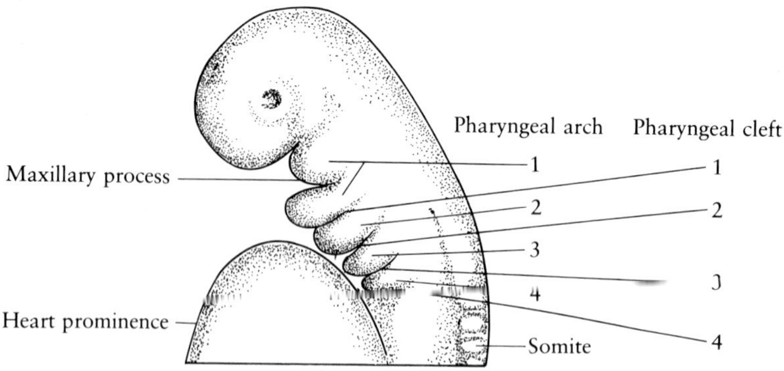

Figure 7-1. Pharyngeal arches

are also numbered correspondingly to the clefts (Figure 7-2) in lower vertebrates; for example, in fish, the pharyngeal clefts and pouches communicate with each other by the breaking down of the intervening membrane to form gill slits. In human beings, however, this communication is never established, and the intervening membrane between the first pharyngeal cleft and pouch later gives rise to the tympanic membrane.

An important landmark is the buccopharyngeal membrane, which lies between the first pharyngeal arch and ventral to the

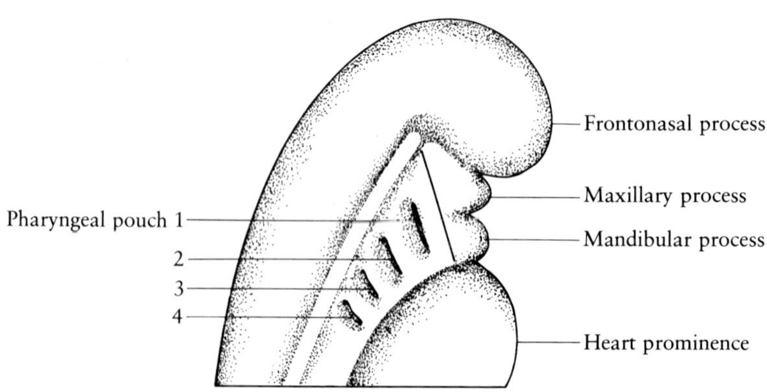

Figure 7-2. Pharyngeal pouches

rapidly developing head end of the embryo. Rupture of this membrane marks the beginning of development of the derivatives of the pharyngeal apparatus. In addition to the pharyngeal apparatus, the frontonasal process also contributes to the formation of the structures of the face and neck region. For the sake of clarity, the developmental processes will be divided up into several sections, although it must be kept in mind that the separate sections are developing simultaneously.

Pharyngeal Arches

Each pharyngeal arch has four components associated with it. These are a cartilaginous component, a muscular component, a nerve, and a blood vessel. The derivatives of the various components of the individual pharyngeal arches are summarized in Table X. In addition, the structural role of each arch is described below.

FIRST PHARYNGEAL ARCH

The first pharyngeal arch consists of two parts: (1) a cranial part, called the maxillary process, forms the maxilla and plays a major role in the development of the upper part of the face (discussed later), and (2) the caudal part, called the mandibular process, grows ventrally to fuse with the mandibular process of the other side and form the mandible. The cartilaginous component of this arch is a transitory structure known as Meckel's cartilage. The dorsal part of this cartilage degenerates, except for a small portion that gives rise to the malleus and incus. The middle portion becomes fibrous, forming the sphenomandibular ligament. A small part of the cartilage adjacent to the malleus also becomes fibrous and is known as the anterior ligament of the malleus. The ventral part of Meckel's cartilage degenerates, and the mandible is formed secondarily through membraneous ossification.

SECOND PHARYNGEAL ARCH

The second pharyngeal arch is known as the hyoid arch, and its cartilage is called Reichert's cartilage. This cartilage gives rise to several structures. The dorsal end remains cartilaginous and

ally, obliteration is incomplete, and a space (a cervical cyst) may persist deep to the skin in the neck region.

Pharyngeal Pouches

FIRST PHARYNGEAL POUCH

The ventral portion of the first pharyngeal pouch elongates to form the pharyngotympanic tube. Its dorsal end enlarges to form the tympanic cavity enclosing the ossicles (Figure 7-4). The lining at the end of this pouch forms the medial surfaces of the tympanic membrane.

SECOND PHARYNGEAL POUCH

Most of the second pouch is obliterated. The epithelium proliferates and penetrates the surrounding mesenchyme. These buds are later invaded by lymphoid tissue to form the palatine tonsils (Figure 7-4).

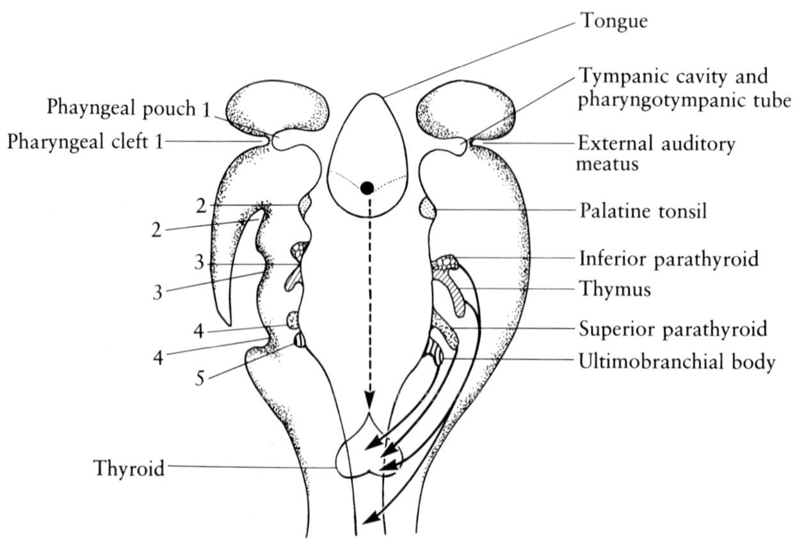

Figure 7-4. Derivatives of pharyngeal clefts and pouches

THIRD PHARYNGEAL POUCH

Two structures are derived from the third pouch. The dorsal part differentiates into the inferior parathyroid gland, and the ventral part forms the thymus (Figure 7-4). Migration of the thymus into the thoracic cavity draws the inferior parathyroid gland downward to its final location on the thyroid gland.

FOURTH PHARYNGEAL POUCH

The fourth pouch gives rise to the superior parathyroid glands, which also migrate downward to lodge in the thyroid gland.

FIFTH PHARYNGEAL POUCH

The fifth pouch, which is vestigial, is thought to give rise to the ultimobranchial body that forms the C cells of the thyroid gland.

FLOOR OF THE PHARYNX

The ventral ends of the pharyngeal arches fuse in the midline and form the floor of the pharynx. The tongue, thyroid gland, and two salivary glands are derivatives of this area.

Tongue

The tongue develops from several primordia, which explains its curious innervation by several nerves. For ease of description, the embryology of the tongue will be broken down into a discussion of the development of its component parts.

BODY OF THE TONGUE (ANTERIOR TWO THIRDS)

The body is formed from the tuberculum impar and lateral lingual swellings. The tuberculum impar is a little mound of tissue located at the junction of the fused mandibular processes (Figure 7-5). The mesenchyme lateral to the tuberculum impar is also elevated and forms the lateral lingual swellings. These primordia are first seen at the end of the fourth week of development. As development proceeds, the lateral lingual swellings overgrow the tuberculum impar to form the body of the tongue.

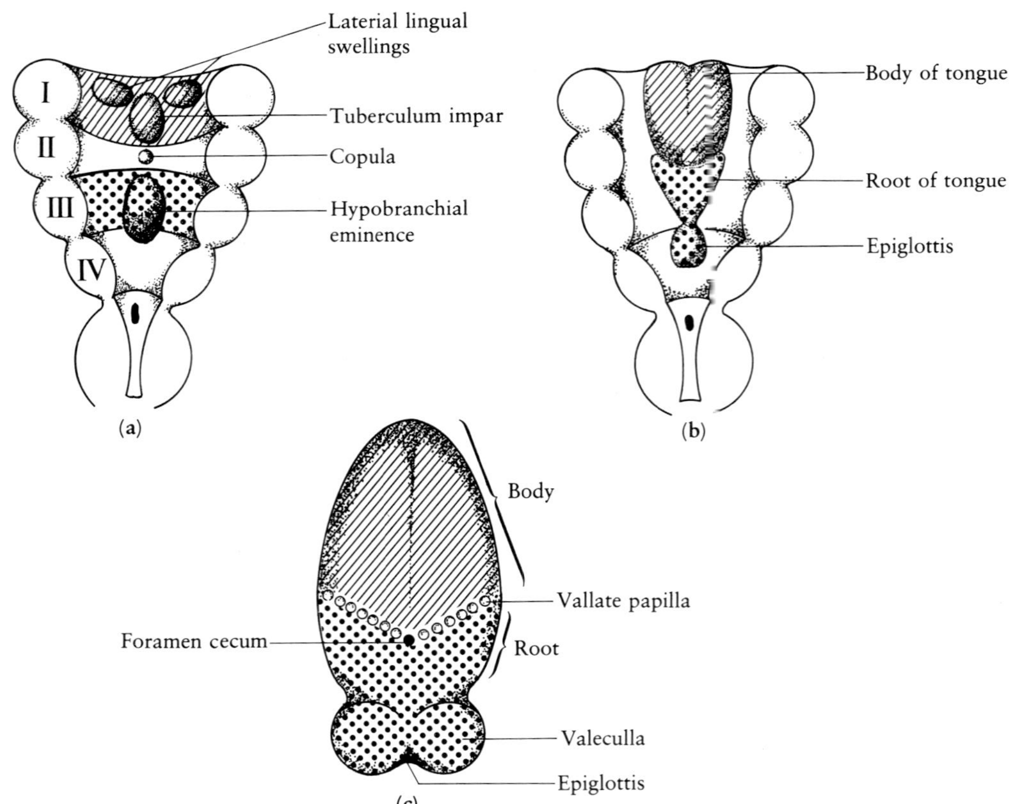

Figure 7-5. Development of the tongue: **A** Week 4; **B** week 5; **C** adult

ROOT OF THE TONGUE (POSTERIOR ONE THIRD)

The copula is a transitory swelling of mesenchyme that arises between the ventral ends of the second pharyngeal arch (Figure 7-5). The hypobranchial eminence is located between the ventral ends of the third and fourth pharyngeal arches. As the tongue develops, the anterior half of the hypobranchial eminence overgrows the copula and forms the root of the tongue. The root of the tongue joins the body at the V-shaped sulcus terminalis.

MUSCLES OF THE TONGUE

The muscles of the tongue apparently arise from the occipital somites and invade the epithelial covering of the tongue. As a result, all the muscles of the tongue except for the palatoglossus are innervated by the hypoglossal nerve. A reexamination of the section on the tongue given in Chapter 5 will assist in the understanding of the complex pattern of innervation of this organ.

Epiglottis

The epiglottis is derived from the posterior half of the hypobranchial eminence. As the anterior half migrates forward during the development of the tongue, a depression appears that becomes deepened as a result of the backward migration of the posterior half of the hypobranchial eminence. This depression is known as the glossoepiglottic fossa, which is subsequently divided into the valleculae by the median glossoepiglottic fold. Elastic cartilage develops within the tissue derived from the posterior half of the hypobranchial eminence and forms the epiglottis.

Thyroid Gland

The thyroid originates as a downgrowth from the floor of the mouth. The diverticulum develops between the first and second arches and is marked in the adult tongue by the foramen cecum. The distal end of the diverticulum soon becomes bi-lobed and will give rise to the lobes of the thyroid gland. The original stalk cavitates and is known as the thyroglossal duct. By the seventh week, the thyroid gland has reached its final site in front of the trachea. The thyroglossal duct usually degenerates and becomes fragmented, so that the attachment to the floor of the mouth is severed. Occasionally, however, the thyroglossal duct may remain patent and serve as a site where food and bacteria may lodge, leading to subsequent infection.

Salivary Glands

SUBMANDIBULAR GLAND

The submandibular gland arises from an epithelial ridge lateral to the tongue. The posterior part of the ridge separates and grows backward and ventral into the surrounding mesenchyme. It enlarges and branches to form the body of the gland. The cranial stalk is maintained as the submandibular duct.

SUBLINGUAL GLAND

The sublingual gland is derived from a series of solid epithelial buds located between the mandible and tongue. These buds enlarge in situ to form the sublingual gland, and its numerous ducts open in the floor of the mouth lateral to the tongue.

PAROTID GLAND

Although not a true derivative of the floor of the mouth, as a salivary gland, the parotid must be included for the sake of completeness. This gland appears during the sixth week as an epithelial outgrowth at the lateral part of the angle of the mouth. The advancing bud branches and develops into the gland, which comes to lie anterior to the external auditory meatus. The original stalk cavitates to form the parotid duct.

Other minor oral glands such as the buccal, labial, and palatine glands arise in situ from epithelial buds.

DEVELOPMENT OF THE FACE

The primordia responsible for the formation of the face are the frontonasal process and the first and second pharyngeal arches (Figure 7-6). The maxillary process grows ventrally to fuse with the frontonasal process, thereby forming the upper part of the

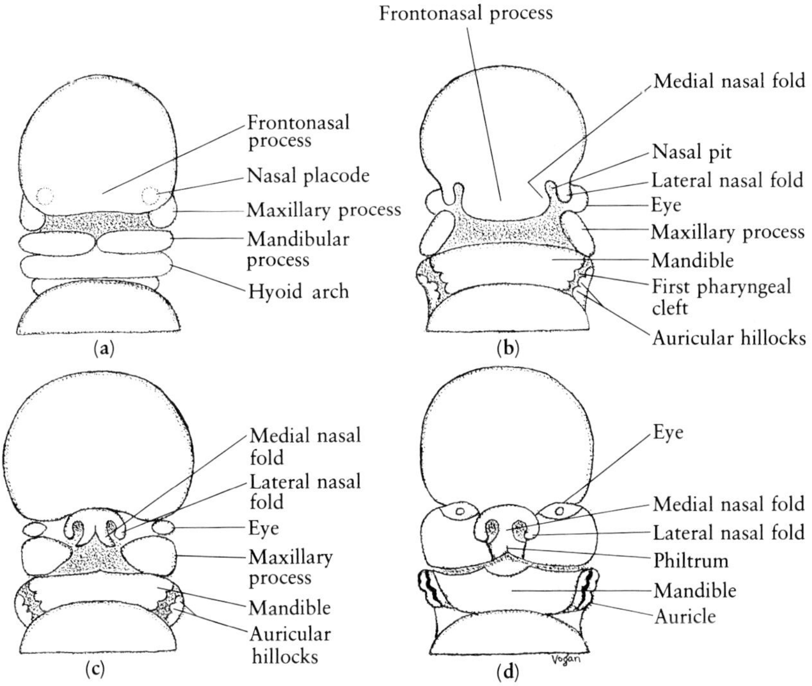

Figure 7-6. Development of the face: **A** 4 weeks, **B** 5 weeks; **C** 6 weeks; **D** 7 weeks

face. The lower jaw is formed from the mandibular process, as previously mentioned. However, the formation of the nose and primary palate are deeply involved in the development of this area and will be discussed at this time. Again, it should be emphasized that the various structures are all developing simultaneously. For the sake of clarity, however, we will study the formation of one structure at a time.

Nose and Primary Palate

Two thickenings known as nasal placodes appear on the anterior end of the embryo above the buccopharyngeal membrane. These thickenings soon become depressed as a result of the proliferation of the tissue surrounding them. The depressions are known as nasal pits and the surrounding tissue as the medial and lateral nasal folds (Figure 7-6). Further deepening of the nasal pits form the nasal sacs. The medial portions of each nasal sac fuses, as do the two medial nasal processes. Proliferation of mesoderm from the frontonasal process extends dorsally to infiltrate this area, giving rise to the primitive palate and part of the nasal septum. Rupture of the posterior end of the nasal sac establishes communication between the anterior opening of the nasal cavity (anterior nares) and the common oronasal cavity. Later, when separation of the nasal cavity is completed by the formation of the secondary palate (to be described below) the conchae will develop as elevations on the lateral nasal walls. In later fetal and ealry postnatal life, small outgrowths of the lateral nasal wall invade the maxilla, frontal, ethmoid, and sphenoid bones to form the paranasal sinuses.

Upper Part of the Face

Concurrent with the development of the nasal cavities, the maxillary processes fuse with the frontonasal process. The line of fusion runs from the medial margin of the eye, down the lateral margin of the nose, and along the lateral edge of the philtrum (Figure 7-6). The philtrum is derived from the frontonasal process. The nasolacrimal duct arises as a solid cord of cells at the line of fusion of the maxilla and frontonasal process. It extends from the medial margin of the eye to the lower part of the nasal cavity. Toward the end of gestation, this cord of cells cavitates to form the duct that empties into the inferior meatus of the nasal cavity. Occasionally, cavitation of the nasolacrimal duct may not be completed until after birth.

Formation of the Palate

Subsequent to its external fusion with the frontonasal process, two projections develop from the medial part of each maxillary process. These processes are called palatal processes. The shelves attempt to grow horizontally toward each other, but because of the bulbous nature of the developing tongue, which fills the common oronasal cavity at this stage, they are forced to turn vertically. With further growth of the mandible, the tongue becomes relatively smaller, and the palatal processes reorient themselves horizontally. Fusion of the two shelves in the midline is then possible. This fusion begins just in front of the middle portion of the shelves and proceeds anteriorly and posteriorly. Anteriorly the palatal processes fuse with the primary palate and superiorly with the midline nasal septum. Fusion of the palate is complete by the seventh week of development. During later development, the anterior part of the palate becomes ossified as the hard palate. The posterior part beyond the nasal septum becomes the fibromuscular soft palate.

Many of the clefts in the palate and face are thought to result from improper fusion of the component structures.

DEVELOPMENT OF THE EAR

The anatomical division of the ear into the external, middle and internal ear corresponds to the fact that each of these parts arise from different primordia. The embryological development of each division will be discussed separately.

External Ear

During the fifth week of development, three hillocks of tissue develop on either side of the first pharyngeal cleft. These hillocks are derived from the first and second pharyngeal arches. Subsequent development leads to the formation of the *auricle,* with the derivatives of the second pharyngeal arch making the major contributions.

The *external auditory meatus* is formed from the deepening of the first pharyngeal cleft (as described earlier). The lateral cartilaginous portion is continuous with and derived from the cartilage framework of the auricle.

The *tympanic membrane* is a trilaminar membrane that arises at the junction of the first pharyngeal cleft and pouch. Its lateral surface is covered with skin derived from the external auditory meatus. There is an intervening layer of fibrous connective tissue, and its medial surface is covered by mucosa from the tympanic cavity.

Middle Ear (Tympanic Cavity)

The tympanic cavity develops from the dorsal end of the first pharyngeal pouch. It expands to enclose and surround the developing ossicles, at the same time investing them with an epithelial covering. Further posterior expansion of the tympanic cavity gives rise to the aditus, which leads into the mastoid antrum and air cells.

Internal Ear

During the fourth week of development, a thickening of the surface ectoderm adjacent to the developing hindbrain is recognized as the otic placode. This otic placode deepends as an otic pit and eventually becomes cut off from the surface ectoderm as the otic vesicle. The otic vesicle gives rise to the membranous labyrinth. This vesicle looks somewhat like an inverted pear with a small diverticulum. The diverticulum grows out to form the endolymphatic sac and duct. The wider part of the vesicle become differentiated in such a way that three flattened sacs are observed at rights angles to each other. The central part of each sac degenerates, leading to the formation of three tubes—the semicircular ducts—at right angles to each other (Figure 7-7). Meanwhile, the narrow end of the sac elongates and begins to coil to form the cochlear duct. The area between the semicircular ducts and cochlear duct differentiates into two sacs, the utricle and saccule, and remains connected to the endolymphatic duct. As differentiation of the membranous laryrinth progresses, the mesenchyme surrounding the ducts differentiate into cartilage. In the region of the semicircular ducts, there is a partial breakdown of the cartilage to form the perilymphatic space surrounding the ducts. Around the cochlear duct, breakdown of the cartilage gives rise to the scala vestibuli and scala tympani. The utricle and saccule are housed in a common chamber, the vestibule, in which they

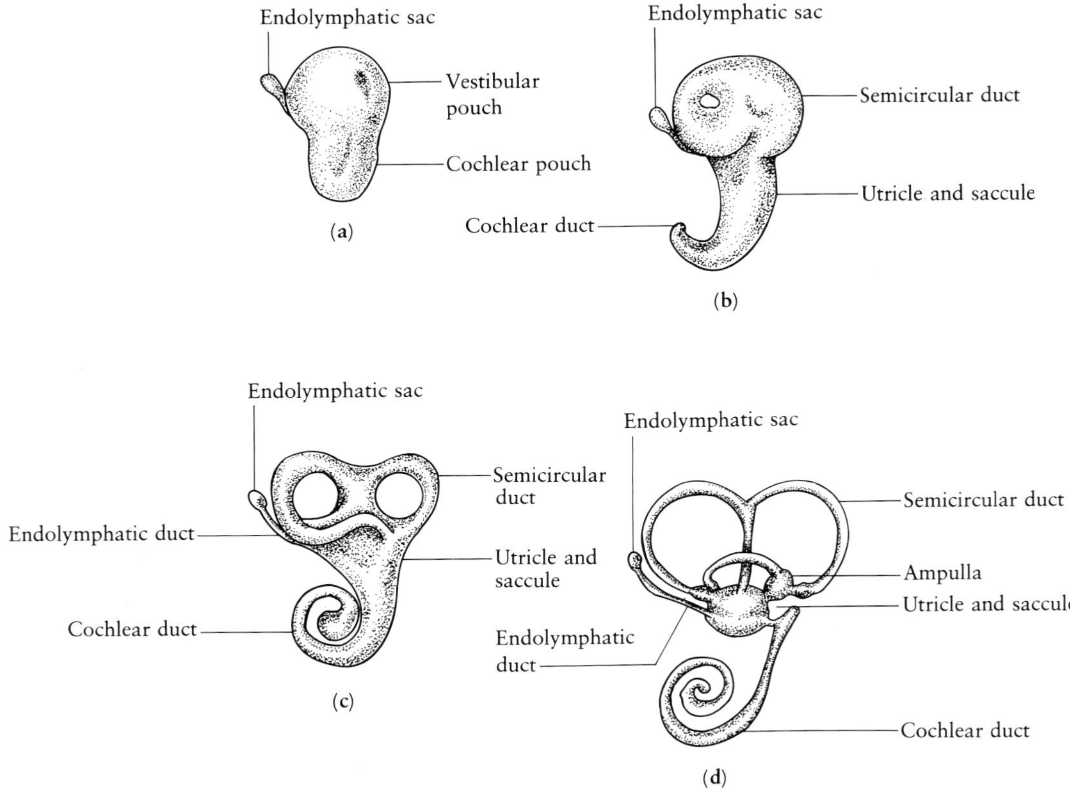

Figure 7-7. Development of the membranous labyrinth: **A** 5 weeks; **B** 6 weeks; **C** 7 weeks; **D** 8weeks

are also surrounded by the perilymphatic space. Ossification of the cartilaginous capsule occurs later in development The cellular organ of Corti differentiates from the thickened floor of the cochlear duct (scala media) adjacent to the scala tympani.

REVIEW QUESTIONS

1. Describe the development of the structures derived from the pharyngeal arches.
2. Describe the development of the structures derived from the pharyngeal pouches.
3. Describe the development of the face.
4. Describe the development of the tongue.
5. Describe the development of the ear.

SUGGESTED READINGS

Hamilton, W. J., Boyd, J. D., and Mossman, H. W. *Human Embryology,* 3rd ed. W. Hepper & Sons, Cambridge, 1964, pp. 203–230, 377–381.

Moore, K. L. *The Developing Human,* 2nd ed. W.B. Saunders Co., Philadelphia, 1977, pp. 156–187, 366–374.

Glossary

Abduction [L. *abductus,* led away] Movement away from the central axis.

Acupuncture [acu + L. *punctura,* prick] The insertion of needles at specific points to produce analgesia.

Adduction [L. *ad,* to; *ducere,* to lead] Movement toward the central axis.

Alveolus (ălvē'ölŭs) [L. *alveolus,* small pit] A small depression or pit.

Ampulla (ămpŭl'a) [L. *ampulla,* flask] A flasklike enlargement.

Anastomosis (ănăs'tömō'sis) [Gk. *ana,* up; *stoma,* mouth] Network of blood vessels or nerves.

Anatomy [Gk. *ana,* up; *tome,* cutting] The science that deals with the study of the human body.

Aperture [L. *apertura,* opening] An orifice or opening.

Arteriole [L. *arteriola,* small artery] A small artery.

Artery [L. *arteria,* artery]. A vessel that carries blood away from the heart.

Arthrodia (âr thrō de'ăh) [Gk. *arthrodia,* articulation] A type of synovial joint.

Articulation [L. *articulus,* joint] A place at which bones are joined together.

Aryepiglottic fold (ary'epi'glot'tic). Upper border of vestibular membranes.

Arytenoid (ăr'ite'noid) [Gk. *arytaina,* pitcher; *eidos,* form] A pair of small cartilages of the larynx articulating with the lamina of the cricoid cartilage.

Auricle (ôr'ĭkl) [L. *auricula,* small ear) A lobulated appendage.

Basilar [L. *basilaris,* base] As in basilar membrane—the membrane that forms the base of the organ of Corti.

Belly The fleshly contractile part of a muscle.

Bifurcation [L. *bi,* two; *furca,* forks] The site where a single structure divides into two parts.

Bolus [Gk. *bolos,* lump] A mass of food ready to be swallowed.

Bone [A.S. *bon,* bone] Dense connective tissue with mineral salts in ground substance.

Bronchiole (brŏng'kĭōl) [Gk. *brongchos,* windpipe] A small subdivision of the bronchus.

Bronchus (brŏng'kŭs) [Gk, *brongchos,* windpipe] One of the major divisions of the trachea.

Buccal (bŭk'ăl) [L. *bucca,* cheek] Pertaining to the cheek.

Bursa (bŭr'să) [L. *bursa,* purse] A fluid-filled connective tissue sac located around joints at points of function or pressure.

Canaliculus (kănălĭk'ūlŭs) [L. *canaliculus,* small channel] A small opening or pore through which another structure passes.

Capsule [L. *capsula,* little box] The covering enclosing an organ.

Cartilage (kâr'tĭlĕj) [L. *cartilago,* cartilage] Dense connective tissue, somewhat flexible.

Cementum (sēĕnt'ŭm) [L. *caementum,* mortar] Covering of root of tooth.

Ceruminous (sĕrū'mĕnŭs) [L. *cera,* wax] Usually refers to glands that secrete a waxy substance.

Cervical [L. *cervix,* neck] Pertaining to the neck.

Choana (kō'ănă) [Gk. *choanae,* funnel] Funnel-shaped opening—posterior nares.

Cochlea (kŏk'lēă) [Gk. *kochlias,* snail] Coiled part of inner ear that houses organ of hearing.

Concha (kŏng'kă) [Gk. *kongche,* shell] A structure resembling the shell of a snail.

Condyle (kŏn'dīl) [Gk. *konkylos,* knuckle] A rounded process on a bone for articulation.

Copula (kop'u lah) [L.] A connecting part.

Corniculate (kôrnĭk'ŭlāt) [L. *cornu,* horn] The name of two small cartilages on apex of the arytenoid cartilages.

Cornu (kôr'nū) [l. *cornu,* horn] Horn or arm of a structure.

Cranial [Gk. *kranion,* skull] Referring to the head end of the body.

Cricoid (krīk'oid) [Gk. *krikos,* ring; *eidos,* form] Ringlike cartilage of larynx.

Crista galli (krĭs'tă gal'e) [L. *crista,* crest; *gallus,* chicken] A projection on the superior surface of the ethmoid bone.

Cuneiform (kūnē'ĭfôrm) [L. *cuneus,* wedge; *forma,* shape] Usually refers to two small cartilages embedded in aryepiglottic folds.

Cupula (ku'pu lah) [L.] Inverted cup or dome-shaped cap.

Cyst [Gr. *kystus,* sac] A sac containing a liquid material.

Deciduous (dē sĭd'ūŭs) [L. *de,* away; *cadere,* to fall] Lost at the end of growth period, e.g., deciduous teeth.

Deglutition (dē gloot ĭsh'ŭn) [L. *deglutire,* to swallow down] The act of swallowing.

Dentine (dĕn'tīne) [L. *dens,* tooth] The chief substance of a tooth.

Diaphragm [Gk. *diaphragma,* midriff] A muscuoltendinous partition separating the thoracic and abdominal cavities.

Diverticulum (di vertik'u lum) [L. *divertere,* to turn aside] A pouch or sac.

Duct [L. *ducere,* to lead] A tube that carries a substance produced by an organ.

Ectoderm [Gk. *ektos,* outside; *derma,* skin] The outermost of the three primary germ layers of the embryo.

Eminence A prominence or projection on a bone.

Enamel The hard material covering the tooth.

Endoderm [Gk. *endon,* within; *derma,* skin] The innermost of the three primary germ layers of the embryo.

Endolymph [Gk. *endon,* inside; L. *lympha,* water] The fluid formed within the membranous layrinth.

Endosteum (ĕndŏs'tēŭm) [Gk. *endon,* inside; *osteon,* bone] The internal lining of the cavity of a bone.

Epiglottis (ĕp'ĭgloŏt'ĭs) [Gk. *epi,* upon; *glotta,* tongue] The flap of cartilage that covers the entrance to the larynx.

Epithelial (ĕp'ĭ thē'lĭăl) [Gk. *epi,* upon; *thale,* nipple] Refers to cellular layer that lines or covers a structure.

Expiration [L. *ex,* out; *spirare,* to breath] The act of breathing out.

Facet [L. *facies,* face] A smooth surface or depression for articulation.

Fascia (fash'e ah) [L. *fascia,* band] A sheet or band of fibrous tissue.

Fauces (faw'sēz) [L. *faux,* narrow passage] The passage from the oral cavity to the pharynx.

Fenestra cochleae (fĕnĕs'tră) [L. *fenestra,* window] The round window in the medial wall of the middle ear that is covered by the secondary tympanic membrane.

Fenestra vetibuli (fĕnĕs'tră) [L. *fenestra,* window] The oval window in the medial wall of the middle ear that lodges the foot of the stapes.

Fibrous joints [L. *fibra,* band] Refers to joints in which the bones are held together by fibrous connective tissue.

Folia (fo'le ah) [L. *folium,* leaf] Leaflike.

Foramen (fŏră'mĕn) [L. *foramen,* opening] A hole permitting the passage of blood vessels or nerves.

Fossa (fŏs'ă) [L. *fossa,* ditch] A shallow depression.

Fovea (fō'vēă) [L. *fovea,* pit] A small depression or pit.

Frenulum (fren'u lum) [L. *fraenum,* bridle] A small fold of mucous membrane.

Ganglion [Gk. *gangglion,* little tumor] Collection of neurons outside of the central nervous system.

Geniculate (je nik'u lāt) [L. *genu,* knee] Bent like a knee.

Gingiva (jĭnjĭ'vă) [L. *gingivae,* gums] The mucous membrane covering the alveolar bone in which the teeth are embedded.

Ginglymus (jin'glī mus) [Gk. *ginglymos,* hinge] A synovial joint with a hingelike action.

Sesamoid (ses amoid) [Gk. *sesamon* sesame; *eidos,* form] Seedlike bone.

Sheath [Gk. *theke,* case] Connective tissue tube surrounding a structure.

Somite (so'mīt) [Gk. *soma,* body] Blocklike mesoderm arranged alongside the neural tube in an embryo.

Subdural [L. *sub,* under; *durus,* hard] Space between the dura mater and the skull.

Suture [L. *sutura,* seam] Immovable articulation between two bones.

Sympathetic [Gk. *sym,* with; *pathos,* feeling] Thoracolumbar portion of the autonomic nervous system.

Symphysis (sĭm̆fĭsĭs) [Gk. *symphysis,* growing together] A joint in which two bones are united by cartilage.

Synchondrosis (sĭn kŏndrō'sĭs) [Gk. *syn,* with; *chondros,* cartilage] A cartilaginous joint.

Syndesmosis (sĭn dĕsmō'sĭs) [Gk. *syndesmos,* ligament] A fibrous joint.

Synovial (sĭnō'vĭal) [Ck. *syn,* with; L. *ovum,* egg] Pertaining to synovia—a viscous lubricating fluid found in joint cavities (synovial fluid).

Tendon [L. *tendere,* to stretch] A connective tissue cord that connects a muscle to bone.

Thymus [Gk. *thymos*] *A ductless gland located in the upper thoracic cavity.*

Thyroid [Gk. *thyra,* door; *eidos,* form] An endocrine gland located in the neck.

Tonsil [L. *tonsilla,* tonsil] Aggregates of lymphoid follicles.

Trabecula (trăbĕk'ūlă) [L. *trabecula,* little beam] Connective tissue septa extending into an enclosed cavity.

Trachea [L. *trachia,*windpipe] The cartilaginous tube descending from the larynx to the bronchi.

Trigone (trīgōn) [Gk. *trigonon,* triangle] A triangular area.

Trochlea (trŏk'lēă) [Gk. *trochilia,* pulley] A pulleylike structure.

Trochoid (tro'koid) [Gk.] Pulleylike (see above).

Tubercle (tū'bërk×el) [L. *tuberculum,* small hump] Small, rounded eminence.

Tympanic (tĭm păn'ĭk) [Gk. *tympanum,* drum] Pertaining to the middle ear; tympanic membrane.

Utricle (ū'trikl) [L. *utriculus,* small bag] The larger chamber of the vetibular portion of the membranous labyrinth.

Uvula (ū'vūlă) [L. *uva,* grape] A small median projection of the soft palate.

Vallecula (val lek'u lah) [L. *valles,* a hollow] A depression between the base of the tongue and the epiglottis.

Ventricle [L. *ventriculus,* belly] Cavity or chamber.

Vestibule [L. *vestibulum,* passage] A passageway.

Vestigial [L. *vestigia,* a trace] Rudimentary or relic.

Index

References to illustrations are in italic type.